365 Days of Soap Making

I0423433

365 Soap Making Recipes for 365 Days

By Coral James

Table of Contents

February

Heart-Shaped Soaps
Carnation Soap Cubes
Nutty Liquid Shampoo
Healthy Hair Shampoo Bar
Strawberries and Champagne Bubble Bath
Ring-Around-The-Rosy Soap
Rose Petal Sugar Scrub
Snowflake Shimmer Soap
Dandy Donut Soap
Berry dish Washing Soap
Cherry Blossom Laundry Soap
Lilac Lover's Foot Suds
Peachy Keen Soap
Loofah Soap
Almond and Apricot Soap Bar
Reusing Herbs For Soap Making – Tea Method
Jasmine Foaming Hand Soap
Homemade Dryer Sheets
Beautifying Face Wash
Hot Chocolate Soap
Homemade Acne Soap
Cloth Diaper Detergent
Purr-fect Cat Cleanser
Natural Diaper Cream
DIY Deodorant
Man Soap
Vanilla Soap Squares
Raspberry Bar Soap
Fruity Hair Mask

March

Heavy-Duty Toilet Scrub
Daily Cleansing Toilet Spray
Tub and Shower Mildew Spray
Tub and Shower Scrub
Daily Cleansing Shower Spray
General Household Disinfectant
Air Cleanser
Spring-Inspired Hand Soap

All-Purpose Kitchen Cleaner
Cutting Board Cleaner
Oven Cleanser
Garbage Disposal Cleaner
Miracle Microwave Cleaner
Super Sink Drain Unclogger
Pan De-Greaser
Cast Iron Pan Scrub
Dandy Dishwasher Detergent
Spring-Inspired Dish Soap
Fantastic Fridge Cleaner
Extreme Disinfectant Cleanser
Spring-Inspired Laundry Soap
Spring-Inspired Fabric Softener
Sweet-Smelling Laundry Sachet
Non-Toxic Bleach Alternative for Laundry
Fancy Floor Cleaner
DIY Window Cleaner
Fantastic Furniture Polish
Silver Cleaner
Carpet Deodorizer
Spring-Inspired Linen Spray
Spring-Inspired Dog Wash

April

Awaken Your Inner Goddess Soap Bar
Warm Sunny Day Soap Bar
Rejuvenating Spring Night Soap Bar
Manly Spring Soap Bar
Sweet Spring Breeze Soap Bar
Women's Secret Soap Bar
Lemon Lover's Spring Soap Bar
Spring Spa Soap Bar
Citrus Breeze Spring Soap Bar
Herbal Citrus Soap Bar
Spring Supernatural Soap Bar
I Need Grounding Soap Bar
Man With a Gentle Hand Soap Bar
Antibacterial Coconut Oil Hand Soap
Black Facial Soap
Natural Plant-Based Elderflower Facewash
Raw Honey Face Cleanser

Kickin' Kiwi Face Mask
Baby Carrot Soap Cake
Beatifying Hair Mask
Heavenly Honey, Yogurt, and Olive Oil Hair Mask
Butterfly-Shaped Soaps
Homemade Citrus Body Scrub
Soap isn't only for your body. You've got to keep you smile clean, too.
Try this DIY toothpaste.
DIY Mouth Rinse
Coconut and Lime Soap
Orange Peel and Rosemary Soap
Jasmine Soap
Rose Petal Foot Soak

May

Dog Paw Wash
Soothing Pet Bath Wipes
Fruit Bowl Soap
Bacon Fat Soap
Monkey Soap
Car Wash Soap
DIY Shoe Soap
Dragon Soap
Mother's Soap
No-Rinse Shampoo Spray
Dry Shampoo
Berry Minty Foot Soap
Buttercream Bar Soap
Chocolate Chip Cookie Soap
Mango Mint Shampoo Bar
Good Morning Sunshine Soap
Lavender Fields and Chamomile Dreams Soap
Sweet Baby Sudsy Soak
Herbal Milk Bath for Wee Ones
Cleansing Anti-Septic Tincture
Tea Rose Enchantment Bar Soap
Carrot Vegetable Soap Bar
Lemon Olive Complexion Bar
Neem Oil Soap
Vitalizing Vitamin Soap
English Countryside Soap
Glowing Body Polish

Vanilla Honey Oatmeal Bar
Cucumber Ivy Mint Magic Soap Bar
Morning Coffee and Cream Sudz Bar
Super Sudsy Sea Sponge Soap

June

Calamine Lotion Soap Bar
Choco Choco Crisp Soap Bar
Mega Citrus Sunshine Shampoo Bar
Simple Coconut Vanilla Layer Soap Bar
Berry Blast Smoothie Soap
Sultry Hair Rinse
Ginger Citrus Dry Shampoo
Honey Almond Face Polish
Gentleman's After Shave
Milky Shea Butter Soap
Intense Moisture Bar
Peppermint Foot Scrub
Summer-Inspired Salt Scrub
Perfectly Pear Soap Bar
Bubble Gum Kid-Approved Soap Bar
Bug Repellant Soap
Canola Oil Soap
Fabulous Flax Oil Soap
Precious Moments Soap
Awesome Bar Soap Recipe
Honey Carrot Sweet Soap
Lazy Day Summer Soap Recipe
Pampering Soap Bar recipe
Peppermint Perk Soap Bar
Big, Beautiful Bubbles Soap Bar
Tantalizing Tea Bar
Mother Earth Soap
Fancy English-Inspired Soap
French Citrus Soap Bar
Honey Bee Baby Soap

July

Skin Loving Soap Bar
Glorious Lemon Rosemary Soap Bar

Love Your Body Soap
Butter Lover's Bodacious Bod Soap
Love Your Face Bar
Leftover Soap Madness!
Milk and Honey Baby Bar
One with Nature Soap
Herbal Soap Scrolls
Orange Mocha Garden Bars
Orange Mocha Dream Fragrance Oil Recipe:
Get Relaxed Soap Bar
Soap for My Summertime Lover
Rosy Complexion Bar
Oceania Soap
Exfoliating Honey Oatmeal Bath Bar
Azuki Bean Cucumber Kokum Skin Nourishing Soap Bar
Boozy Bay Rum Soap Bar
Super Sweet Honey Almond Body Bar
Exfoliating Milk and Honey Bee Soap
All About Milk Based Soap
Minty Chocolate Soap
Grandpa's Old-Fashioned Goat's Milk Soap
Silky Smooth Shampoo Bar
Sweet Summer Rays Soap Bar
Simply Shea Butter Soap
Sow Your Wild Oats Soap Bar
White Zinfandel Soap
Sunny Complexion Soap Bar
Dead Sea Rejuvenating Face Mask
Enchanted Beauty Facial Love
Mango Mint Shampoo Bar

August

Two Lovers Aphrodisiac Bath Oil
Cleansing Bath Salts
Fizzy Bath Bombs
Soapy Bath Syrup
Little Girl's Pink Bath Fairy Dust
Little Boys' Blue Bath Gnome Dust
Chocolate Bath Cream
End of Summer Chocolate Bath Fizzers
Pretty Skin Flower Bath Salts
Flower Child Herbal Hippie Soak

Honey Body Wash
Tub Tea
End of Summer Bath Soak
Bath Candy
Silky Bath Soak
Raspberry Passion Sugar Scrub
White Chocolate and strawberry Sugar Scrub
Hygienic Body Powder
Hot Weather Cooling Foot Powder
Summer Soap Jellies
Lemony Goat's Milk Soap Bars
Kids' Bath Crayons
Cherry Soda Cupcake Cuties
Succulent tangerine Soap
Vanilla Bean Oatmeal Bar
Vanilla Rose Soap Bar
Honey Lemon Tea Bar
Floral Bouquet Bars
Red Rooibos Tea Bar
Baby Powder Scent Bar
Honey Suckle Soap Bar
Honey Olive Bar

September

Apricot Yum Yum Soap
Argan Oil Soap
Awapuhi Sea Berry Soap
Adorable Baby Shower Gift Soap
Bastille Soap
Brewsky Bar Soap
Blackberry Sage Soap
Scrumptious Blueberry Cheesecake Soap Bars
Warm and Sunny Calendula Soap
Creamy Calendula Swirl Soap Bar
Carmel and Custard Creamy Soap
Bunny Bliss Carrot Soap
Classic Cleo Heavy Cream Soap
Lickity Split Lemonade Soap
Soap Frosting
Whirly Swirly Soap
Creamy Coconut Soap Bars
Doggy Delight 'Poo

Energizing Soap Bar
Frantic Fruit Frenzy Soap
Soothing Avocado Soap
Supermarket Soap Recipe
Lotus Blossom Sea Salt Soap
Psychedelic Hemp Soap
Wholesome Hot Fudge Brownie Soap
Hunting Trip Super Soap
Lovely Lady Lavender Soap
Girlfriends Soap
Luscious Lime Soap
Mystic Mango Soap Bars

October

Pumpkin Puree Soap
Nutmeg Butter Soap
Gone Batty Soap
Jack-O-Lantern Soap
Candy Corn Soap
Monster Soap
Alien Soap
Body Parts Scary Soap
Icky Eyeball Soap
Vampire Fangs Soap
Creepy Bugs Soap
Slithering Snake Soap
Pumpkin Pie Bars
Apple Pie Milk Bath
Apple Spice Soap
Cool, Autumn's Night Soap
Red Wine Soap
Gorgeous Man Soap
Sweet Orange Chili Pepper Soap
Yummy Wheatgrass Soap
Lemon Lime Bundt Cake Soap
Beet Root Facial Soap
Candy Apple Soap
Carrot Cupcake Soap
Cinnamon Bun Soap
Cammy Clay Soap
Chocolate Cream Cheese Cupcake Soap
Ghost Soap

Count Dracula's Dentures
Freshly Fallen Leaves Soap
Monster Boogers Soap

November

Star Anise Soap Bars
Cinnamon Pumpkin Paradise Soap
Rustic Soap Bars
Warm Ginger Patchouli Soap Bars
November Moustache Soap
Soap on a Rope Pumpkins
Shimmering Fall Layer Soap
Save Face Cleansing Bars
Cranberry Seed Soap Bars
"The Leaves of Fall" Soap Bars
Licorice Soap Cubes
Pumpkin Smiles Soap
Honeycomb Soap
Carmel Apple Soap
Bath Whip Frosting
Gnome Soap
Giving Thanks Soap Bars
Honey Ale Soap
Dainty Little Leaves
Glitter Cut-Out Autumn Soap
Stenciled Glitter Autumn Soap
Realistic Pumpkin Soaps
Thanksgiving Turkey Soap
Mother's Love Soap
Red Lychee Soap
Ducky Soap
Pilgrim Soap
Cornucopia Soap
Mayflower Soap
Sunflower Soap

December

Christmas Candy Soap
Christmas Tree Soap
Christmas Ornament Soap

Introduction

Have you ever wondered how you can make your own soaps, washes, scrubs, and other cleaning agents for both the body and home? This may come as a shock to you, but running to the supermarket to purchase soap isn't always necessary. In fact, you can create an abundance of soaps from your very own home using ingredients that you most likely have on-hand in your pantry. It really is that simple, and this book is going to teach you how.

365 Days of Soap making for Beginners is a book dedicated to the new soap maker. Our recipes aren't overly complex, and they teach you how to make simple soap concoctions using safe instructions. Not only will you be able to make your own soap after reading this book, but you'll have fun doing it in the process. You'll find a recipe for each day of the year.

Enjoy making a variety of soaps that use non-toxic materials like herbs, essential oils, and castile soap. So many soaps on the market today are filled with chemicals, carcinogens, and other toxic substances that can be harmful to you, your family, pets, and the environment. Take a stand against these chemicals and start making your own soaps and cleaning products today.

Now, let's get started!

Basic Soap Making Methods

This book will give you a large variety of recipes for making soaps. Here are a few basic methods that you can apply to some of them.

Cold Process Soap Making

"Cover your work area with newspaper. Put your gloves and other protective wear on. Measure your water into the quart canning jar. Have a spoon ready. Measure your lye. Slowly pour the lye into the water, stirring as you go. Stand back while you stir to avoid the fumes. When the water starts to clear, you can allow it to sit while you move to the next step.

*In the pint jar, add your oils together. They should just make a pint. Heat in a microwave for about a minute, or place the jar of oils in a pan of water to heat. Check the temperature of your oils – it should be about 120° or so. Your lye should have come down by then to about 120°. Wait for both to cool somewhere **between 95° and 105°.** This is critical for soap making. Too low and it'll come together quickly, but be coarse and crumbly.*

*When both the lye and oils are at the right temperature, pour the oils into a mixing bowl. **Slowly** add the lye, stirring until it's all mixed. **Stir by hand for a full 5 minutes.** It's very important to get as much* *of the lye in contact with as much of the soap as possible. After about 5 minutes, you can keep stirring, or you can use an immersion blender. The soap mixture will lighten in color and become thick. When it looks like vanilla pudding it's at "trace" and you're good to go.*

Add your herbs, essential oils or other additions at this point. Stir thoroughly to combine. Pour the mixture into mold(s) and cover with plastic wrap. Set in an old towel and wrap it up. This will keep the residual heat in and start the saponification process. Saponification is the process of the base ingredients becoming soap.

After 24-hours, check your soap. If it's still warm or soft, allow it to sit another 12-24 hour. When it's cold and firm, turn it out onto a piece of parchment paper or baking rack. If using a loaf pan as your mold, cut into bars at this point. Allow soap to cure for 4 weeks or so. Be sure to turn it over once a week to expose all the sides to air (which is not necessary if using a baking rack). For a DIY soap drying rack, I took an old potato chip rack and slid cardboard fabric bolts (from a fabric store) through the rungs.

When your soap is fully cured, wrap it in wax paper or keep it in an airtight container. Handmade soap creates its own glycerin, which is a humectant, pulling moisture from the air. It should be

wrapped to keep it from attracting dust and de-
bris with the moisture."

Source: http://www.diynatural.com/

Hot Process Soap Making

"Hot process soap is an interesting take on the
cold process method. The simple explanation is
that you take all your ingredients, and add them
to a pot (that is then placed over a heat source,
such as a stove) and frequently stir until the soap
goes through various stages. The excess water is
evaporated off, and the soap is ready to use once
cooled."

Source: Debra Maslowski at http://teachsoap.com/

Melt and Pour Soap

"Technically, all handmade soap is "Glycerin
Soap." In many commercial soaps, all the extra
glycerin (formed naturally by the cold process
soap making method) is harvested out. Thus, all
handmade soap is glycerin rich (since handmade
soap makers don't harvest out glycerin in their
soap).

In today's market, the term "Glycerin Soap" is
commonly used to refer to clear soap. Generally,
the clear soap has extra glycerin added to it to
produce a very nourishing, moisturizing bar.
Glycerin is a "humectant." It draws moisture to

itself; the theory is that if you wash with glycerin soap, a thin layer of glycerin will remain, drawing moisture to your skin.

Clear soap base can be purchased in large blocks to be melted down, colored and fragranced, and placed into molds (or used to make loaves of soap be sliced). This type of soap is called "Melt and Pour" and the artistry of melt and pour is called "Soap Casting." Melt and Pour soap making are gaining in popularity because of its ease of use. There are no significant safety measures (other than basic common sense – don't put your hand in the hot soap, don't cut your finger off with the knife, etc.) needed for soap casting. Children can do it. It's a great outlet for creative types.

You can also make clear soap from scratch. This method involves all the aspects of cold process soap making, but takes it a few steps further by adding alcohol for clarity and glycerin and sugar mix to suspend and enhance the clarity. It is a dangerous process because of the alcohol vapors. If you wish to make clear soap (which will not melt down like melt and pour – it's one pour only soap), please read "Making Transparent Soap" by Catherine Failor. This is an excellent resource for anyone wishing to make clear soap from scratch."

Source: http://teachsoap.com/

Safely Using Lye

Lye is a material used in almost all soaps. However, if not handled properly, using lye can be disastrous. To avoid accidently burns to the skin, lungs, and mucous membranes, always take precautions when using lye.

- Wear proper safety gear

- Mix lye in a well-ventilated area

- ALWAYS add lye to water and NEVER water to lye

- Use a lye appropriate mixing vessel

- Store lye appropriately

- Immediately rinse lye from your skin if direct contact occurs. Seek out medical attention.

To learn more about the dangers of lye and how to keep yourself safe when using it, please visit: https://www.soapqueen.com/bath-and-body-tutorials/tips-and-tricks/back-to-basics-lye-safety-guide/

January

January marks the beginning of a new year. Bring this new year in with a bang by making a variety of your own soaps and cleansers. In many parts of the world, January is a very cold, winter month. Skin and hair tend to be very dry. In this chapter, we'll focus on moisturizing soaps as well as soaps that contain natural ingredients that ward of germs and illnesses. Here's to soft skin and healthy bodies during the month of January!

January 1

Basic Hand and Body Soap Recipe

- 2/3 c. refined coconut oil
- 2/3 c. extra virgin olive oil
- 2/3 c. almond oil (or any other oil that you prefer)
- ¼ c. lye
- ¾ c. purified cool water

Use the Cold Process Soap Making method for this recipe.

January 2

Aloe Vera Soap

- 15 oz. refined coconut oil
- 13.5 oz. extra virgin olive oil
- 10.5 oz. lard
- 2.5 oz. organic shea butter

- 10 oz. aloe vera gel and water puree

- 6.5 oz. lye

- 10 oz. purified water

Use the Cold Process Soap Making method for this recipe.

January 3

Anise Soap

- ¼ c. Anise seeds

- ¼ c. lard

- ¾ c. tallow

- ¼ c. vegetable oil

- ½ c. cold filtered water

- 2 tbsps. lye

Heat the 1/4 c. of tallow or lard until melted. Add anise seed and simmer over lowest heat for half an hour. If you have a wood stove, set on back all day. Leave to solidify for a few hours or overnight, then melt again and strain seeds. Add enough additional melted tallow or lard to the strained anise fat to measure 3/4 cup. Add vegetable oil and set aside to cool.

Stir lye into cold water until thoroughly dissolved and set aside to cool. Grease molds liberally with **petroleum jelly**. When lye and fat are lukewarm, pour lye into fat, stirring constantly. Continue to stir until the mixture has saponified and is as thick as creamed honey. Pour into molds. Approximate Yield: 12 oz. hard bar soap.

Source: http://www.soaprecipes101.com/

January 4

Warm Honey Soap

This recipe is great for hot showers on cold winter days. Honey is also known for it's antibacterial properties.

- 48% beef tallow, rendered
- 25% extra virgin olive oil
- 20% coconut oil
- 5% castor oil
- 2% beeswax
- Lye
- Distilled water
- 4% essential oil blend of citronella and lemongrass
- 3% raw honey

Slowly add the lye to the water, mix until fully dissolved and set aside to cool. Melt the beeswax in a double boiler until liquid. Heat the remaining oils and tallow and stir until fully dissolved and even in texture and color.

When lye & fats are lukewarm, pour lye slowly into fat, stirring until thick and creamy. Add warm wax mixture in a thin stream, beating vigorously to disperse evenly. Add honey and essential oils. Pour into molds.

Source: http://www.soaprecipes101.com/

January 5

Winter Rose Soap

- 28 oz. refined coconut oil

- 42 oz. extra virgin olive oil

- 12 oz. sunflower oil

- 11.73 oz. Lye

- 26 oz. strained rose petal infusion (create a tea)

- At trace, stir in 1 tablespoon each of rosehip seed oil, jojoba oil and melted shea butter. (optional, makes a higher superfatted bar)

- Also at trace, add a few teaspoons geranium essential oil.

Use the Cold Process Soap Making method for this recipe.

January 6

Winter Weather Wonder Shampoo

When Old Man Winter is wreaking havoc on your hair, fight back with this moisture-rich shampoo recipe.

- ¼ c. spring water

- ¼ c. castile soap

- ½ tsp. light vegetable oil

Mix all ingredients together in a measuring cup, and pour into a clean squeeze bottle. Shampoo hair as normal.

January 7

Winter Weather Wonder Conditioner

Follow up with this amazing moisture-rich conditioner after using Winter Weather Wonder Shampoo.

- 1 c. spring water

- 2 tbsp. apple cider vinegar

- 10 drops of lavender, sandalwood, or geranium essential oil

Mix all ingredients together in an 8 oz. squeeze bottle. Shake before using. Use conditioner after shampooing and allow to sit for at least 5 minutes before rinsing.

January 8

Moisturizing Pet Soap

It's not just humans who get dry, itchy skin during the winter months, your pet suffers, too! Try this homemade pet soap recipe to soothe your dog's dry skin.

- 1 c. oatmeal

- ½ c. baking soda

- 1 qt. warm water

Using a food processor or blender, grind the oatmeal until it reaches a flour consistency. Place the oatmeal powder into a bowl and carefully stir in the baking soda. Next, add the warm water to the mixture and stir until thoroughly mixed. Suds up your dog as you normally would with this fabulous soap.

January 9

Winter Foot Soap Soak

When your feet are feeling frigid due to plummeting winter temperatures, this sudsy DIY foot soak is sure to warm them up.

- ¼ c. lemon juice
- ¼ c. milk
- 3 tbsps. extra virgin olive oil
- 1 tbsp. castile soap
- 1/8 tsp. cinnamon

Place all ingredients in a large basin and add hot warm. Give the solution a stir with your hand, and allow your feet to soak for as long as you like.

January 10

Happy Winter Skin Facial Soap

Is your face dried out due to frosty winter air? Treat yourself to this moisture-rich facial soap.

- 2 apple slices, peeled
- ½ c. plain yogurt
- ½ c. tbsp. olive oil
- ½ tbsp. raw honey

Blend all ingredients in a food processor or blender until smooth and creamy. Massage soap onto skin and allow to sit for 5-minutes. Rinse with warm water.

January 11

Moisturizing Honey Shower Wash

- 2/3 c. castile soap
- ¼ c. raw honey
- 2 tsps. grapeseed oil
- 1 tsp. vitamin E oil
- 50 – 60 drops vanilla essential oil

Place all ingredients into a recycled shampoo or body wash container and shake vigorously. Squirt onto a washcloth or loofah.

January 12

Homemade Dish Soap

- 1 ¾ c. boiling water
- 1 tbsp. borax
- 1 tbsp. grated Ivory or Castile bar soap
- 15 – 20 drops of orange or lemon essential oil

Heat water until boiling. Next, add the borax and grated bar soap to a medium bowl. Then, pour the boiled water over the top of the soap mixture. Whisk until the soap is dissolved. Allow the mixture to cool for about 8 hours, stirring every now and then. Transfer the dish soap to a squirt bottle and add in the essential oil. Shake well to combine.

January 13

Homemade Laundry Soap

- 1 cup washing soda
- 1 cup borax
- 1 bar of Fels-Naptha soap, grated
- 50 drops of your favorite essential oil

Mix all ingredients together in a bowl or jar and cover with an airtight lid. Use 1 – 2 tbsps. Per a load of laundry. This detergent is HE safe.

January 14

Cold Weather Liquid Hand Soap

Keep those hands from chapping in January's brutal breeze with this DIY liquid hand soap.

- ½ c. castile soap
- ½ c. distilled water
- 1 tbsp. vitamin E oil
- 1 tbsp. sweet almond oil
- 15 drops tea tree essential oil
- 5 – 10 drops lavender or peppermint essential oil

Add water, liquid castile soap, and oils to a mason jar. Cap the jar and shake until all ingredients are evenly incorporated. Replace the lid with a pump dispenser.

January 15

Goats Milk Soap

- 9.52 oz. refined coconut oil
- 11.11 oz. olive oil
- 1.59 oz. castor oil
- 6.35 oz. palm oil
- 3.18 oz. shea butter
- 7.58 oz. distilled water
- 3.53 oz. goats milk
- 4.5 oz. lye

Follow the Cold Process Soap Making method.

January 16

Exfoliating Coffee and Cinnamon Soap

- 6 ½ c. olive oil
- 7/8 c. lye
- 2 ½ c. water
- 1 – 5 tbsps. coffee grounds
- 20 drops of cinnamon leaf essential oil
- A few sprinkles of ground cinnamon

Follow the Cold Process Soap Making method.

January 17

Foaming Shave Soap

- 1/4 c. natural aloe vera gel
- 1/4 c. liquid castile soap
- 1 tbsp. olive or almond oil
- 1/4 c. warm distilled water
- Vitamin E or grapefruit seed extract
- Essential oils for fragrance
- 8 oz. or larger foaming soap bottle

Mix all ingredients together in a foamer bottle and shake gently to incorporate.

January 18

Creamy Shave Butter Soap

- ¼ c. Coconut oil
- 2 -3 tbsps. cocoa butter
- ¼ c. raw honey
- 1 tbsp. kaolin clay
- 2 tsp. baking soda
- ¼ c. liquid castile soap
- Vitamin E

Melt the oil and cocoa butter in a double boiler. Remove pan from heat and add the remaining ingredients. Whisk for several minutes. Transfer the shave butter soap to a glass jar and cover with a lid.

January 19

Sleepy Time Soap for Kids

- ½ c. Castile soap
- ½ c. distilled water
- 2 tbsps. fractionated coconut oil
- 1 tsp. vegetable glycerin
- 10 drops lavender essential oil

Add water to a glass jar or soap dispenser followed by the castile soap. Next, add the remaining ingredients. Cover the jar with a lid and shake vigorously to evenly mix.

January 20

Homemade Bath Paint Soap

Make bath time fun with homemade bath paint soap!

- ¼ c. shampoo, hand soap, or body wash
- ¼ c. corn starch
- 1-2 tbsps. water
- 3-4 drops food coloring

Combine the cornstarch, shampoo, and food coloring in a bowl. Next, add the water by ½ tbsp. Increments until the paint reaches the desired consistency. Store in plastic containers with lids.

January 21

Baby Boo Shampoo

- ¼ c. Castile soap

- 2 tbsps. sweet almond oil

- 1 tbsp. organic aloe vera gel

- 2 drops chamomile essential oil

Add all ingredients to a glass jar and stir. Place a lid on the jar and store.

January 22

Creamy Coconut Milk Hair Wash

- ½ c. Liquid castile soap

- ¼ c. canned coconut milk

- ¼ c. raw honey

- 2 tbsps. fractionated coconut oil

- 1 tbsp. vitamin E oil

- 10 drops each of lemon, lavender, tea tree, and rosemary essential oils

Mix all ingredients together in a glass container with a lid or an old shampoo bottle and shake to evenly combine. Always shake well before each use.

January 23

Old-Fashioned Pine Tar Soap

This nostalgic DIY soap is the answer to dry, itchy skin, eczema, dandruff, and psoriasis.

- 13.5 oz. lard
- 13.5 oz. olive oil
- 8.2 oz. palm kernel oil
- 5.8 oz. sunflower oil
- 7.2 oz. pine tar
- 5.9 oz. lye
- 15.8 oz. water
- 2 oz. lavender, tea tree, eucalyptus, and Siberian fir essential oil blend
- 1 tbsp. sugar added to the water for the lye solution, before you add the lye

Follow the Cold Process Soap Making method.

January 24

Peppermint and Rosemary Soap

- 15 oz. olive oil
- 13 oz. coconut oil
- 2.6 oz. castor oil
- 16 oz. distilled water
- 6.2 oz. lye

- 0.8 oz. peppermint essential oil

- 0.8 rosemary essential oil

- 0.4 oz. sage essential oil

- ¼ oz. spirulina

- 1 oz. dried peppermint leaves

Follow the Cold Process Soap Making method.

January 25

Homemade Warm Vanilla Body Scrub

- 1 c. brown sugar

- ½ c. granulated white sugar

- ½ c. coconut oil

- 1 tbsp. vanilla extract

- 2 vitamin E capsules

- 1 tbsp. castile soap

Combine all ingredients in a large bowl and mix well. Store in an airtight container.

January 26

Winter Blues Bubble Bath

Relax in a tub filled with uplifting scents with this marvelous bubble bath recipe.

- 1 c. unscented castile soap

- ½ c. vegetable glycerin

- 2 tbsps. water
- 15 drops of your favorite essential oil

Combine first 3 ingredients together in a glass container. Add the essential oil and stir. When ready to use, add ¼ to ½ cup under running tub water.

January 27

Beautiful Body Suds

Use this body wash to uplift your mood and get your mind thinking about Spring.

- ½ c. unscented castile soap
- 4 tbsps. vegetable glycerin
- 3 tbsps. fractionated coconut oil
- 10 drops lemon essential oil

Combine the first 3 ingredients in a glass bowl followed by the essential oil. Stir well. Pour body wash into an 8 oz. soap dispenser bottle and use during shower or bath time.

January 28

Keep Your Mouth Clean DIY Rinse

Soap isn't only for your body. Keep the germs at bay with this all-natural mouth rinse. Don't worry, it tastes great!

- 2 tbsps. water
- ½ tsp. baking soda

- 2 drops peppermint essential oil
- 1 drop patchouli essential oil

Combine the baking soda and water in a small container, followed by the essential oils. Mix well and swish in your mouth for 1 minutes before spitting.

January 29

Hot Press Crock Pot Soap

- Crisco — 9.6 ounces or 272.155 grams
- Olive oil OR olive oil pomace — 9.6 ounces or 272.155 grams
- Lard — 6.4 ounces or 181.437 grams
- Coconut oil (76-degree melt point) — 6.4 ounces or 181.437 grams
- Distilled water — 12.16 ounces or 344.73 grams
- Lye — 4.463 ounces or 126.524 grams

Follow the Hot Process Soap Making Method, but use your Crock Pot as your heat source.

Learn more about this recipe here:
http://chickensintheroad.com/house/crafts/hot-process-soap-in-a-crock-pot/

January 30

Late January Laundry Bar Soap

- 10.8 oz. refined coconut oil

- 18 0z. palm oil

- 7.2 oz. soybean oil

- 5.2 oz. lye

- 11 oz. distilled water

At trace:

- .75 oz. borax

- .4 oz. lime essential oil

Follow the Cold Process Soap Making Method.

January 31

DIY Liquid Laundry Softener

- 1-gallon white vinegar

- 30-40 drops of your favorite essential oil

Add the essential oil to a gallon jug of white vinegar, cap, and shake. Use ¼ c. Per load. Safe for HE washers.

February

Ah, the season of love. February is a month of passion, intimacy, and lots of loving soap bubbles in your bathtub. Cupid is sure to point his arrow directly at you this month as you handcraft beautiful soaps for the ones you love.

February 1

Heart-Shaped Soaps

Give your sweetie a passion-filled bath experience with these cute heart-shaped soaps.

- Melt-and-pour transparent soap block in red or pink
- Heart-shaped soap molds
- Essential or fragrance oils of your choice

Cut soap block into small cubes. Bring a few cups to boil in a double boiler. Turn down the heat and allow water to simmer. Add the soap cubes. Stir gently until melted. Remove the soap from the heat and allow to cool slightly before adding in oils. Pour soap into heart-shaped molds and let harden for two hours.

February 2

Carnation Soap Cubes

- 32 oz. Shea Melt and Pour Base
- 32. oz. Aloe Melt and Pour Base

- Liquid Violet

- Lagoon Green Jojoba Beads

- Purple Jojoba Beads

- Sierra Sky Jojoba Beads

- 9 Cube Soap Silicone Mold

- Carnation Fragrance Oil

To start, mix 2 tbsps. of each color of jojoba bead in a glass mixing bowl and set aside. Next, cut 16 oz. of Shea melt and pour base. Add the base to a glass bowl and heat soap in the microwave until it melts, stirring every 10 seconds. Now, add the fragrance oil to the melted soap and mix. Allow the soap to cool to around 125-130 degrees before adding the beads. Stir constantly. When the soap has cooled, add two tbsps. Of the jojoba bead mixture and mix. Fill soap molds half full with the concoction. Use the alcohol to pop any air bubbles. Cut 16 oz. of Aloe Melt and Pour Base and melt. Add .5 oz. Carnation Fragrance Oil and 1 teaspoon of the Liquid Violet color. Stir well. Melt 16 oz. of Shea Melt and Pour, and repeat steps 2 – 4. Spray the purple soap with isopropyl alcohol before you pour to help the layers stick together. Fill the cavities until they are about 3/4 of the way full. Spray with alcohol again. Allow the soap to fully harden for 1 to 2 hours before unmolding.

Source: http://teachsoap.com/

February 3

Nutty Liquid Shampoo

Give the goofball in your life this nutty shampoo for Valentine's Day.

- 5 Soap Nuts

- 3 c. water

- 5 drops lavender essential oil

Place the soap nuts in a muslin bag. Place the bag into a medium saucepan with 2 cups of the water and bring to a boil. Reduce heat and allow to simmer for 20 minutes. Add the remaining cup of water and simmer for an additional 10 minutes. Remove the pot from the heat and allow to cook. Squeeze the bag until it suds. Rinse with cool water and squeeze into the pan again. Store the shampoo in a glass jar in the refrigerator.

February 4

Healthy Hair Shampoo Bar

- 10 ounces' olive oil (34.5 percent)

- 8 ounces' coconut oil (27.5 percent)

- 5 ounces' sunflower oil (17 percent)

- 4 ounces' castor oil (14 percent)

- 2 ounces' jojoba oil (7 percent)

- 10 ounces distilled water (or cool herbal tea)

- 3.91 ounces' lye

Use the Hot Process Soap Making Method.

February 5

Strawberries and Champagne Bubble Bath

- 1-gallon castile soap or liquid suspension soap base

- 2.56 oz. strawberries and champagne fragrance oil
- 2 oz. red food coloring
- 3 tbsps. iridescent cosmetic glitter

Pour the liquid soap inti a glass vessel. Add 1 tsp. of glitter. Add drops of food coloring to reach the desired shade. Add 10 ml. of fragrance oil and stir. Pour into bottles. Repeat process until you've used up all ingredients.

February 6

Ring-Around-The-Rosy Soap

- Clear suspension soap base
- Dried flowers of your choice
- Soap mold
- Rose and Lavender essential oils
- Beet juice

Cut suspension soap into pieces and slowly melt over medium heat using the double boiler method. Once melted, stir in essential oils and remove from heat. Add beet juice for a colorant. Press flower petals into the bottom of the soap mold and pour the soap on top. Allow to harden for several hours before removing from soap molds.

February 7

Rose Petal Sugar Scrub

- 1 cup dried rose petals
- 2 cups white sugar

- 2/3 cups coconut oil
- 68 drops geranium essential oil

Place rose petals into a blende or food processor and pulse until they are tiny flakes. Combine the crushed petals with the remaining ingredients and store in a glass jar.

February 8

Snowflake Shimmer Soap

Use these winter-themed soaps every time you bathe on a cold day.

- Organic Glycerin Soap Base
- Snowflake Silicone Mold
- Coconut Oil
- Granulated White Sugar
- Blue Soap Colorant
- Cosmetic Shimmer Pearl Powder and Glitter Powder

Combine ½ pound of soap base with 3 tbsps. Coconut oil in a glass bowl. Melt the ingredients in the microwave in 20-second intervals, stirring well each time. Next, stir in 1 tbsp. of glitter powder, 1 tbsp. Colorant, and 1 cup sugar. Transfer the soap to the mold and allow to harden for about an hour before removing.

February 9

Dandy Donut Soap

- Clear glycerin soap base

- Silicone donut mold

- Gold and wine soap colorant

- Cupcake fragrance oil

- Rainbow sprinkles

Place rainbow sprinkles into the bottom of each donut mold. Next, cut the soap base into cubes and place into a glass bowl. Microwave for 20-30 seconds. Stir the soap and microwave again for another 10-15 second. Once completely melted, add the a few drops of wine colorant to the soap and stir. Pour the pink soap into the donut molds. Allow to cool for 15 minutes. Repeat the entire process again only using the gold colorant. Pour soap on top of the pink soap and allow to harden before unmolding.

February 10

Berry dish Washing Soap

- 16 oz. castile soap

- 10 drops juniper berry essential oil

- 5 drops red food coloring

Place all ingredients into a glass jar and mix well. Place a pump-style lid onto the jar and enjoy.

February 11

Cherry Blossom Laundry Soap

- 1 cup washing soda

- 1 cup borax

- 1 bar grated Ivory soap

- 1 tbsps. cherry blossom fragrance oil

Add all ingredients to a glass jar and mix well. Use 1 tbsp. per a load of laundry. HE safe.

February 12

Lilac Lover's Foot Suds

- 1 c. dry milk

- ½ c. Epsom salts

- ¼ c. liquid castile soap

- ½ tbsp. lilac fragrance oil

Mix all ingredients together in a bowl and add to a basin of warm water. Soak feet for as long as you like. This recipe can also be used as a body scrub.

February 13

Peachy Keen Soap

- 4-ounce Soap pure white and unscented

- 1/4 cup Milk powder

- 1/4 cup Distilled water

- 1 tbsp. Almond oil

- 1/8 tsp Peach fragrance oil

- 1 drop Orange food coloring

Use the Melt-And-Pour Soap making Method.

February 14

Loofah Soap

- 30 oz. glycerin soap base
- .9 0z. white tea and ginger fragrance oil
- 20 drops orange liquid soap colorant
- 5-inch loofah

Place loofah into a round soap mold. Follow the Melt-And-Pour Soap making Method.

February 15

Almond and Apricot Soap Bar

- Soap base
- Apricot and almond oil fragrance oil
- Apricot seeds
- Peach-colored soap colorant
- Muffin tin

Follow the Melt-And-Pour Soap making Method.

February 16

Reusing Herbs For Soap Making – Tea Method

There's no sense in throwing away those teabags after you've made yourself a lovely cup of herbal. Simply cut the teabag open and empty the herbs into a glass jar. Place a lid on the jar and store in the refrigerator until you're ready to make an herbal soap.

February 17

Jasmine Foaming Hand Soap

- 12-ounces of Water
- 2 Tablespoons Liquid Castile Soap
- ½ tsp liquid oil like olive or almond
- 20 drops Jasmine essential oil

Fill a foaming soap dispenser bottle almost to the top with water. Add 2 tbsps. of liquid castile soap to the water. Add in the essential oil. Close the lid and swish mixture to incorporate ingredients.

February 18

Homemade Dryer Sheets

These aren't soap, but they are part of the laundry process so we thought we'd throw them in this book for you. Enjoy!

- Old scraps of clean cloth
- Essential oils of choice
- White vinegar
- Glass jar

Mix 1 cup of white vinegar with 25 drops of essential oil. Place folded cloth scraps into the jar and gently moisten by pushing them down. Place a lid on the jar to store. Use one dryer sheet per a load of laundry.

February 19

Beautifying Face Wash

- ½ c. mashed strawberries
- 1 tbsp. honey

Mix the ingredients together in a bowl until evenly incorporated. Apply the face wash onto the face and massage for about 4 minutes. Rinse with warm water and pat skin dry.

February 20

Hot Chocolate Soap

- 2 tsp whole milk powder
- 2 tsp instant coffee granules
- 1 tbsp. cocoa powder
- 2 tsp vanilla flecks
- 2 tsp ghassoul clay (or other brownish clay)
- 2 tsp French red clay (or other ruddy reddish clay)
- 5g cocoa absolute
- 10g vanilla 10-fold essential oil

Follow the Cold Process Soap Making Method.

February 21

Homemade Acne Soap

Say goodbye to those pesky pimples during the month of love.

- 6.08 ounces of filtered water

- 2.33 ounces Lye

- 6.4 ounces Coconut Oil

- 6.4 ounces Olive Oil

- 3.2 ounces Castor Oil

- 1 tablespoon activated charcoal powder

- 1 tablespoon bentonite clay powder

- 1 ounce of essential oil of choice like tea tree oil or lavender

Follow the Cold Soap Method.

February 22

Cloth Diaper Detergent

- Washing Soda

- Baking Soda

- Oxygen Cleaner

Mix all ingredients together in a container with a tight-fitting lid. Use 1-2 tbsps. of detergent per a load of dirty diapers.

February 23

Purr-fect Cat Cleanser

We all know that cats hate to get wet, so this DIY soap is used in dry form.

- ½ c. arrow root powder

- ¼ baking soda

- 3 drops pet-friendly essential oil

Mix all ingredients together in a glass jar. Sprinkle a tbsp. or two into your palm and massage into the cat's fur.

February 24

Natural Diaper Cream

- ½ c. Coconut oil
- 1 tbsp. calendula flowers
- 1 tbsp. chamomile flowers
- ¼ c. shea butter
- 1 tsp. arrowroot powder

Melt coconut oil using a double boiler method. Add the flowers to the pot and reduce to medium-low and allow mixture to simmer. Once the coconut oil starts to turn yellow, remove pot from heat. Next, carefully strain the flowers out using a cheesecloth. Reserve the coconut oil in a bowl. Next, mix in the shea butter and arrowroot powder using an immersion blender. Store in a glass jar. Use between diaper changes.

February 25

DIY Deodorant

- 1/2 cup coconut oil
- ½ cup baking soda
- 40-60 drops essential oil
- Empty deodorant container

Place coconut oil in a bowl. Mix in the baking soda followed by the essential oils. Store the finished product in an empty deodorant container.

February 26

Man Soap

- Soap base
- Cypress essential oil
- Green-colored soap colorant
- Muffin tin

Follow the Melt-And-Pour Soap making Method.

February 27

Vanilla Soap Squares

- Soap base
- Vanilla fragrance oil
- Grated vanilla bean
- tan-colored soap colorant
- Square soap mold

Follow the Melt-And-Pour Soap making Method.

February 28

Raspberry Bar Soap

- Soap base

- Raspberry fragrance oil

- Pink-colored soap colorant

- Soap molds in the shapes of your choice

Follow the Melt-And-Pour Soap making Method.

February 29

Fruity Hair Mask

- 1 very-ripe banana, mashed

- 1 tsp. almond oil

Mix ingredients together in a bowl and apply to dry hair. Cover head with a shower cap and allow mixture to sit for at least 20 minutes before rinsing. Shampoo and condition as normal.

March

Spring has finally begun! Yay! During this month, we will learn soap making recipes for household cleaners that will help you tackle the beast of winter gunk that's been lurking in your home. Some of these recipes won't be your traditional hot or cold press soap recipes, but are still cleansers, nonetheless. Start spring right with these refreshing everyday soaps to get you and yours sparkling clean and germ-free.

March 1

Heavy-Duty Toilet Scrub

- ½ c. baking soda
- 10 drops tea tree essential oil
- ¼ c. white vinegar

Dump all of the ingredients into the toilet bowl and scrub using a toilet brush. Flush when finished cleaning.

March 2

Daily Cleansing Toilet Spray

- Small spray bottle
- 1 c. white vinegar
- 5 drops lemon or tea tree essential oil

Place all ingredients into the spray bottle, cap, and shake well. Spray onto toilet surface and wipe with a clean cloth.

March 3

Tub and Shower Mildew Spray

- Small spray bottle
- 10 drops lemon essential oil

Add ingredients to the spray bottle, cap, and shake to mix. Spray solution onto offending area and allow to sit for 30-minutes before rinsing with warm water.

March 4

Tub and Shower Scrub

- 1 c. baking soda
- ½ cup castile soap

Mix ingredients together in a bowl and apply to problem areas with a scrub brush to remove tough stains. Rinse with warm water.

March 5

Daily Cleansing Shower Spray

This is a great recipe to use after your daily shower.

- 1 large spray bottle
- 2 c. white distilled vinegar
- 30 drops essential oil of your choice (tea tree or citrus oils work best due to their disinfecting properties)

Mix all ingredients into a large spray bottle, cap, and shake. Use after showering by spraying walls, faucet, and glass slider door (if your shower has one). No need to rinse.

March 6

General Household Disinfectant

- Large spray bottle
- 2 c. water
- 3 tbsps. castile soap
- 20-30 drops tea tree oil

Combine all ingredients into a spray bottle, cap, and shake to incorporate. Use in bathrooms, kitchen, countertops, etc.

March 7

Air Cleanser

It's not only surfaces that need the power of soap. Banish offensive bathroom smells with this quick air freshening recipe.

- Glass jar and lid
- 1 c. baking soda
- 40 drops of your favorite essential oil

Place baking soda and essential oil into the glass jar and mix. Place the lid on the glass jar and poke holes in it. Set the jar in your bathroom to release a pleasant, air-cleansing aroma.

March 8

Spring-Inspired Hand Soap

After all of this bathroom cleaning, you need to keep your hands germ-free, right?

- Pump-style hand soap bottle 9preferably with a foamer lid)
- Enough castile soap to fill container halfway
- Water
- 1-2 drops of Bergamot essential oil

Add Castile oil soap to fill bottle halfway followed by the water. Place the essential oil into the bottle, cap, and shake.

March 9

All-Purpose Kitchen Cleaner

- 1 Large spray bottle
- 2 cups vodka
- 2 cups water
- 10 drops orange essential oil

Add all ingredients to the spray bottle, cap, and shake. Use on countertops, in the microwave, refrigerator, and any kitchen surface that needs to be cleaned.

March 10

Cutting Board Cleaner

- 1 lemon

Cut 1 lemon in half and run it over your cutting board. Allow the juice to sit for 10 minutes before rinsing. For tough stains, scrub the cutting board with course kosher salt. You want to avoid using soap on your wooden cutting board because wood is porous and the essence of the soap will be retained, which could intermingle with your food.

March 11

Oven Cleanser

To clean a stubborn oven, heat it to 125 degrees. Spray All-Purpose Kitchen Cleaner onto stains and caked-on food, followed by salt. Turn the oven off and allow to cool. Use a wet towel to wipe away the gunk. For a bit more elbow grease, scrub with baking soda.

March 12

Garbage Disposal Cleaner

- 1 c. vinegar
- Water

Pour the vinegar into an ice cube tray and top off with water. Once frozen, toss a few cubes down the disposal and run.

March 13

Miracle Microwave Cleaner

- ½ c. white vinegar
- 3 tbsps. lemon juice
- Small microwave-safe cup or bowl

Pour ingredients into the bowl and place into the microwave. Turn the microwave on high-power for 2 minutes. Once finished, remove bowl from the microwave and wipe away gunk with a damp sponge or wash-rag.

March 14

Super Sink Drain Unclogger

Sometimes, food, grease, and other debris get stuck in the drain, and you need to get them out. This recipe will help you do just that.

- 1-gallon boiling water
- ½ c. baking soda
- ½ c. white vinegar
- Pot lid

Pour the baking soda and vinegar down the drain. Wait for them to fizz. Next, dump the boiling water down the drain and cover with a pot lid until fizzing subsides.

March 15

Pan De-Greaser

- Salt
- Scrubber or scouring pad

Pour salt onto the greasy pan and scrub with a brush or scouring pad. Rinse.

March 16

Cast Iron Pan Scrub

Most professional chefs agree that commercially produced soaps are a huge no-no when it comes to cleaning cast iron cookery. We couldn't agree more, which is why you'll love this natural "soap" recipe.

- 3 tbsps. olive oil
- 1 tsp. coarse salt

Add ingredients to the cast iron pan and scrub using a stiff brush. Rinse with hot water when done.

March 17

Dandy Dishwasher Detergent

- 1 c. castile soap
- 1 c. water
- 2 tsps. lemon juice
- 1 qt. glass jar

Add all ingredients to a glass jar and use enough detergent to fill the soap compartment of your dish washer. Fill all other compartments with white vinegar.

March 18

Spring-Inspired Dish Soap

- 1 c. castile soap
- 3 tbsps. water
- 5 drops of your favorite floral essential oil
- Glass jar with a pump top

Mix all ingredients together in the glass jar (or recycled dish washing detergent bottle), cap, and shake.

March 19

Fantastic Fridge Cleaner

- ½ c. baking soda
- 1-gallon hot water

Add ingredients to a bucket and stir. Dip a clean cloth into the solution and wipe down the inside and outside of the refrigerator.

March 20

Extreme Disinfectant Cleanser

Sometimes, a spring illness might arise in your home. In this case, you'll need some additional cleaning-power to ensure all the germs are dead and gone.

- ½ c. baking soda
- 1 tsp. castile soap
- ½ tsp. hydrogen peroxide

Combine all ingredients in a large bowl or basin. Apply the solution to surfaces with a cloth, scrub, and thoroughly rinse with hot water.

March 21

Spring-Inspired Laundry Soap

- 1 bar glycerin soap, finely grated
- 1 c. washing soda
- ½ c. baking soda
- ½ c. citric acid
- ¼ c. coarse salt
- 50 drops of your favorite floral blend of essential oils

Add all ingredients to a large jar and mix together. Cover with an air-tight lid. Use 1-2 tbsps. of detergent per a load of laundry. To prevent detergent from clumping, place tbsps. of white clay into a small, child's sock and tie. Put the sock into the jar of detergent.

March 22

Spring-Inspired Fabric Softener

- 20-30 drops floral scented essential oils
- 1-gallon white vinegar

Close the lid on the white vinegar and shake. Add 1/3 c. of fabric softener per a load of laundry.

March 23

Sweet-Smelling Laundry Sachet

This awesome little laundry sachet makes a wonderful companion to your homemade laundry soap and fabric softener. Simply place the ingredients into the sachet and toss into your dryer.

- Small piece of scrap fabric sewn into a sachet
- 1 ½ c. dried herbs like lavender buds and rose petals

March 24

Non-Toxic Bleach Alternative for Laundry

- ½ c. baking soda
- 1 tsp. castile soap
- ½ tsp. hydrogen peroxide
- 2 tbsps. lemon juice

Add 1/3 c. to the rinse cycle for sparkling colors and gleaming whites.

March 25

Fancy Floor Cleaner

- 1/3 white vinegar
- 2/3 water

Add these ratios to a 1-gallon bucket. Mop floor as you normally would. Make this on an as-needed basis.

March 26

DIY Window Cleaner

- ½ tsp. Castile soap
- 3 tbsps. white vinegar
- 2 c. water
- Small spray bottle

Add all ingredients to the spray bottle, cap, and shake to mix. Spray on windows and wipe streaks away with an old newspaper.

March 27

Fantastic Furniture Polish

- ¼ c. Vinegar
- ¾ c. olive oil

Combine all ingredients in a bowl and use a soft cloth to apply to wooden furniture.

March 28

Silver Cleaner

- 1 bucket
- Aluminum foil
- Boiling water
- 1 c. baking soda
- 1 pinch of salt

Line the bucket or sink with aluminum foil. Place the silverware on top of it. Pour the boiling water over the silverware and add the baking soda and salt. You can use a bit of toothpaste and a soft cloth to clean silverware you do not wish to immerse.

March 29

Carpet Deodorizer

- 1 cup baking soda
- ½ c. ground lavender flowers

Mix all ingredients in a bowl and sprinkle over carpets. Allow to sit for about 20 minutes before vacuuming.

March 30

Spring-Inspired Linen Spray

- 1 small mister bottle
- 1 c. vinegar

- 20-30 drops floral scented essential oil

Mix all ingredients together in the mister bottle, cap, and shake. Mist over linens and furniture for the sweet smells of spring.

March 30

Spring-Inspired Dog Wash

Even Rover needs a spring makeover!

- 1 cup castile soap
- ½ c. vinegar
- 1 drop lemon essential oil

Mix all ingredients together in a glass jar. Dampen your dog's fur with warm water and work the soap into a sudsy lather. Rinse and repeat if necessary.

April

April brings us into the thick of spring days. Now that we've got the house all cleaned up by using the DIY cleansers that we made during the month of March, it's time to pamper our hearts, minds, souls, and bodies with spring-inspired soaps that are scented with essential oils, herbs, and other materials meant to awaken our spirit. This chapter focuses on both hot and cold processed soaps with different essential oil blends.

April 1

Awaken Your Inner Goddess Soap Bar

- 4 parts spearmint essential oil
- 1-part patchouli essential oil

Use all ingredients and instructions listed in the Cold Process Soap Making method.

April 2

Warm Sunny Day Soap Bar

- 2 parts orange essential oil
- 1-part vanilla essential oil

Use all ingredients and instructions listed in the Cold Process Soap Making method.

April 3

Rejuvenating Spring Night Soap Bar

- 1 part lavender essential oil
- 1 part peppermint essential oil

Use all ingredients and instructions listed in the Cold Process Soap Making method.

April 4

Manly Spring Soap Bar

- 1 part patchouli essential oil
- 2 parts bergamot essential oil
- 1 part cedarwood essential oil

Use all ingredients and instructions listed in the Cold Process Soap Making method.

April 5

Sweet Spring Breeze Soap Bar

- 2 parts orange essential oil
- 1 part Use all ingredients and instructions listed in the Cold Process Soap Making method.

Use all ingredients and instructions listed in the Cold Process Soap Making method.

April 6

Women's Secret Soap Bar

Don't let the monthly changes in your body get you down and out. Use this fabulous essential oil soap bar blend for a wonderful retreat of the senses.

- 1 part Clary Sage essential oil
- 2 parts bergamot essential oil
- Red raspberry leaf crushed herbs

Use all ingredients and instructions listed in the Cold Process Soap Making method.

April 7

Lemon Lover's Spring Soap Bar

- 3 parts lemon essential oil
- 2 parts rosemary essential oil
- 1 part cedarwood essential oil

Use all ingredients and instructions listed in the Cold Process Soap Making method.

April 8

Spring Spa Soap Bar

- 3 parts peppermint essential oil
- 2 parts lavender essential oil

- 1 part patchouli essential oil
- .5 parts tea tree essential oil

Use all ingredients and instructions listed in the Cold Process Soap Making method.

April 9

Citrus Breeze Spring Soap Bar

- 3 parts tea tree essential oil
- 3 parts bergamot essential oil
- 2 parts orange essential oil
- 1 part litsea cubea essential oil

Use all ingredients and instructions listed in the Cold Process Soap Making method.

April 10

Herbal Citrus Soap Bar

- 3 parts orange essential oil
- 3 parts rosemary essential oil
- 2 parts lavender essential oil
- 1 part peppermint essential oil
- 1 part litsea cubea essential oil\

Use all ingredients and instructions listed in the Cold Process Soap Making method.

April 11

Spring Supernatural Soap Bar

- 3 parts clary sage essential oil
- 3 parts lemon essential oil
- 2 parts lavender essential oil
- 1 part orange essential oil
- 1 part litsea cubea essential oil

Use all ingredients and instructions listed in the Cold Process Soap Making method.

April 12

I Need Grounding Soap Bar

- 3 parts lemon essential oil
- 3 parts litsea cubeba essential oil
- 2 parts bergamot essential oil
- 1 part peppermint essential oil

Use all ingredients and instructions listed in the Cold Process Soap Making method.

April 13

Man With a Gentle Hand Soap Bar

- 3 parts lavender essential oil
- 2 parts clary sage essential oil

- 2 parts orange essential oil

- 1 part patchouli essential oil

- 1 part cedarwood essential oil

- 1 part litsea cubea essential oil

Use all ingredients and instructions listed in the Cold Process Soap Making method.

April 15

Antibacterial Coconut Oil Hand Soap

- Water

- 2 tablespoons castile soap

- 2 teaspoons fractionated coconut oil

- 15 drops clove essential oil

- 10 drops tea tree oil

- 5 drops each: cinnamon leaf, eucalyptus, peppermint essential oils

Fill an empty foaming soap dispenser ¾ of the way with water. Add the castile remaining ingredients to the bottle, cap, and shake.

April 16

Black Facial Soap

- 1/3 of a bar of African black soap or Dudu osun

- Distilled water

- 3 teaspoons of Grapeseed oil

- 3 teaspoons of raw honey

- 2 teaspoons of ground cinnamon and black pepper

- 2 teaspoons of vegetable glycerin

- 1 teaspoon of vitamin E

- 1/2 a teaspoon or more of guar gum for desired thickness

- Essential oils: Rosemary, bergamot, clove and juniper berry

Cut soap into small chunks and place into a heat resistant jar. Cover soap with boiling water. Leave mixture to sit for at least 3 hours. Next, add the raw honey, cinnamon, black pepper, and grapeseed oil. Then, add the vegetable glycerin, vitamin E, and essential oils and stir. Stir in the guar gum powder to the mixture and whisk thoroughly until thick. Your soap is ready to use!

April 17

Natural Plant-Based Elderflower Facewash

- Handful of soapnuts

- ½ c. soapwort

- 1 c. elderflowers

- ¾ tsp. vegetable glycerin

- Guar gum powder

- A few drops of neroli, sweet orange, and red mandarin essential oils

Allow elderflowers to steep in hot water for 24-hours. Drain the elderflowers and pour infused water into a pot to boil on low heat. Next, add the soapnuts and soapwort. Increase the heat to medium. A soapy substance should start to form. Remove the mixture from the stove and drain. Place the liquid back into the pot and whisk in a half tsp. of guar gum or more followed by the veggie glycerin. Place face wash into desired container and add essential oils.

April 18

Raw Honey Face Cleanser

- Raw tropical rainforest honey – ½ cup

- Manuka honey – 2 tbsps.

- Dried Soapwort bark

- Pure apple cider vinegar – ½ tbsp.

- Bee propolis – ½ tsp

- Frankincense oil – 5 drops

- Lavender oil – 5 drops

- Distilled water

Place ¾ c. dried soapwort into a pan and cover with distilled water and bring to a boil. Reduce heat when mixture becomes soapy and leave to simmer for a few minutes. Remove from heat and strain out bark. Then, add in the propolis and stir. Place the mixture into a container and stir well followed by the ACV and essential oils.

April 19

Kickin' Kiwi Face Mask

This is a great sudsy face mask that leaves your skin feeling gorgeous, smooth, and flawless.

- 1 kiwi fruit
- 2 tbsps. yogurt
- 2 tbsps. raw honey

Place the kiwi into a bowl and mash with a fork. Add the yogurt and honey to the bowl and stir. Spread the mask on your face and allow it to dry for 10-15 minutes. Wash off and follow up with your favorite moisturizer. Your skin will be squeaky clean!

April 20

Baby Carrot Soap Cake

- 4 ounces' carrot puree
- 4 ounces' carrot cooking water (or plain water)
- 1 teaspoon salt (to help with unmolding)
- 3.9 ounces' lye
- 2 ounces Castor Oil (7%)
- 7 ounces Coconut Oil (25%)
- 19 ounces Olive Oil (68%)

Follow the Cold Process Soap Making Method.

April 21

Beatifying Hair Mask

Hair masks don't use traditional soaps but the ingredients included in them provide proper nourishment that cleanses stressed out locks.

- ½ an avocado

- 2 egg yolks

Mix all ingredients together and apply to dry or wet hair. Cover head with a shower cap or towel and allow mask to penetrate tresses for at least 15 minutes before rinsing and washing.

April 22

Heavenly Honey, Yogurt, and Olive Oil Hair Mask

This another recipe that will cleanse your hair and leave it shiny and gorgeous.

- 1 tsp. olive oil

- 1 tbsp. raw honey

- ¼ c. yogurt

Mix all ingredients together and apply to dry or wet hair. Cover head with a shower cap or towel and allow mask to penetrate tresses for at least 15 minutes before rinsing and washing.

April 23

Butterfly-Shaped Soaps

- Melt-and-pour transparent soap block in red or pink

- Butterfly-shaped soap molds

- Essential or fragrance oils of your choice

Cut soap block into small cubes. Bring a few cups to boil in a double boiler. Turn down the heat and allow water to simmer. Add the soap cubes. Stir gently until melted. Remove the soap from the heat and allow to cool slightly before adding in oils. Pour soap into butterfly-shaped molds and let harden for two hours.

April 24

Homemade Citrus Body Scrub

- 2 c. white sugar

- ½ c. coconut oil

- 10 drops citrus blend essential oils

- 2 vitamin E capsules

- 1 tbsp. castile soap

Combine all ingredients in a large bowl and mix well. Store in an airtight container.

April 25

Soap isn't only for your body. You've got to keep you smile clean,

too. Try this DIY toothpaste.

- 2/3 cup baking soda

- 1 tsp fine sea salt

- 1 – 2 tsp peppermint extract or 10-15 drops peppermint essential oil

- Filtered water

Mix all ingredients together and place into a container suitable for dipping your toothbrush into.

April 26

DIY Mouth Rinse

- Small mason jar

- ½ cup filtered or distilled water

- 2 tsp baking soda

- 2 drops tea tree essential oil

- 2 drops peppermint essential oil

Mix all ingredients together and place into a mason jar. Swish 2 tbsps. in your mouth and spit.

April 27

Coconut and Lime Soap

- 15 oz. olive oil

- 13 oz. coconut oil

- 2.6 oz. castor oil

- 16 oz. distilled water

- 6.2 oz. lye

- 0.8 oz. Lime essential oil

- 0.8 Coconut essential oil

- ¼ oz. spirulina

Follow the Cold Process Soap Making method.

April 28

Orange Peel and Rosemary Soap

- 15 oz. olive oil

- 13 oz. almond oil

- 2.6 oz. castor oil

- 16 oz. distilled water

- 6.2 oz. lye

- 0.8 oz. orange essential oil

- 0.8 rosemary essential oil

- 1 oz. orange rind

Follow the Cold Process Soap Making method.

April 29

Jasmine Soap

- 15 oz. olive oil

- 13 oz. coconut oil

- 2.6 oz. castor oil

- 16 oz. distilled water

- 6.2 oz. lye

- 0.8 oz. Jasmine essential oil

Follow the Cold Process Soap Making method.

April 30

Rose Petal Foot Soak

- 1 c. dry milk

- ½ c. Epsom salts

- ¼ c. liquid castile soap

- ½ tbsp. lilac rose oil

- 1 oz. dried rose petals

Mix all ingredients together in a bowl and add to a basin of warm water. Soak feet for as long as you like. This recipe can also be used as a body scrub.

May

April showers bring May Flowers, so they say. What types of flowers and herbs do you have growing in your garden? We're willing to be you have all sorts of nature-inspired goodies in your very own yard that can be used in a variety of soaps and cleaners. April focuses on wrapping up spring and heading into the summer months. In this chapter, you'll find a mixture of soap recipes, pet care products, and even a few oddities.

May 1

Dog Paw Wash

Sometimes Man's best Friend's paw get a bit gritty and grimy. It's best to keep them clean in order to prevent bacterial growth and infection.

- Plastic jug with wide-mouth opening
- Water
- ½ c. castile soap
- 2 drops tea tree oil

Fill the jug halfway with warm water, followed by the soap and essential oil. Swish the solution around to evenly incorporate. Place your pup's paws, one at a time, into the jug to cleanse.

May 2

Soothing Pet Bath Wipes

- Heavy Duty Paper towels or square cloth rags
- Airtight container
- 1/4 Cup Aloe Vera gel
- 1 Vitamin E capsule
- 2 cups hot water
- 2 drops tea tree oil

Separate the paper towels and fold them into rectangles, then fold them over again. Place the towels into the container. Next, pour hot water into a mixing bowl and add the aloe vera gel. Now, break open the vitamin E capsule and pour the liquid into the mixture and whisk for one minute. Add 2 drops of tea tree oil to the mixture. Pour the solution over the paper towels in the container and secure the lid. Turn the container over to moisten the towels.

May 3

Fruit Bowl Soap

- 15 oz. olive oil
- 13 oz. coconut oil
- 2.6 oz. castor oil
- 16 oz. distilled water
- 6.2 oz. lye
- 0.8 oz. strawberry fragrance oil
- 0.8 oz. blueberry fragrance oil
- 0.8 oz. banana fragrance oil

Follow the Cold Process Soap Making method.

May 4

Bacon Fat Soap

Yep, you read that right. Today, you will be taught how to create a bar of soap using the fat off everyone's favorite meat.

- 4 c. liquid bacon fat
- Bacon soap molds
- 4.2 oz. Lye
- 15 drops red and yellow food coloring
- ¾ container for bacon bits for exfoliate

Follow the Hot Process Soap Making method.

May 5

Monkey Soap

- 15 oz. olive oil
- 13 oz. coconut oil
- 2.6 oz. castor oil
- 16 oz. distilled water
- 6.2 oz. lye
- 0.8 oz. banana fragrance oil
- Monkey soap mold

Follow the Cold Process Soap Making method.

May 6

Car Wash Soap

- ½ c. dishwashing soap
- ½ c. baking soda
- 1-gallon warm water

Mix all ingredients together into a bucket. Wash car with solution followed by a rinse with the hose.

May 7

DIY Shoe Soap

- ½ tbsp. Dawn Dish Soap
- 1 tbsp. Baking soda
- 1 tbsp. hydrogen peroxide

Mix together all ingredients in a bowl and apply to shoes with a toothbrush, gently scrubbing away stains and dirt. Rinse shoes with warm water.

May 8

Dragon Soap

- 15 oz. olive oil
- 13 oz. coconut oil
- 2.6 oz. castor oil
- 16 oz. distilled water

- 6.2 oz. lye

- 0.8 oz. Dragon's Blood fragrance oil

- Dragon soap mold

Follow the Cold Process Soap Making method.

May 9

Mother's Soap

- 15 oz. olive oil

- 13 oz. coconut oil

- 2.6 oz. castor oil

- 16 oz. distilled water

- 6.2 oz. lye

- 0.8 oz. clary sage essential oil

- 0.8 oz. neroli essential oil

- Rosemary sprigs

Follow the Cold Process Soap Making method.

May 10

No-Rinse Shampoo Spray

- 1 tbsp. of cornstarch

- 4 tbsp. of water

- 1 tbsp. of rubbing alcohol

- small measuring glass

- Small spray bottle

Mix all ingredients together, and pour into the spray bottle. Shake before each use.

May 11

Dry Shampoo

- ¼ c. corn starch
- 2 tbsps. cocoa powder
- 2-4 drops essential oil of your choice

Place all ingredients into a glass jar, cap, and shake. Brush onto hair roots with a makeup brush and comb through hair.

May 12

Berry Minty Foot Soap

- 9 oz. suspension melt and pour base
- 3/4 tsp. 250 IU vitamin E oil
- 1/4 tsp. raspberry seeds
- 1/4 tsp. blueberry seeds
- Raspberry fragrance oil
- Blueberry fragrance oil
- Peppermint essential oil

Follow the melt and pour soap making method.

May 13

Buttercream Bar Soap

- 4 oz. goats milk melt and pour base

- 1 Tbsp. powdered whole milk

- 1/2 tsp of hydrolyzed silk amino acid

- 8 drops of buttercream fragrance oil

- 8 drops of vanilla fragrance oil

Follow the melt and pour soap making method.

May 14

Chocolate Chip Cookie Soap

- 1 ib. white or clear coconut melt and pour base

- Cocoa powder or brown colorant

- 1 lb. cocoa butter

- 1 tbsp. chocolate fragrance oil

- Small circular soap molds

Follow the melt and pour soap making method.

May 15

Mango Mint Shampoo Bar

- 1 cup grated soap

- 1/2 cup water

- 1/4 cup olive oil

- 1/4 cup castor oil

- 1 t dried crushed peppermint leaves

- 15 drops mango fragrance oil

Use the hot process soap making method.

May 16

Good Morning Sunshine Soap

- 1 cup grated soap

- 1/8 cup safflower oil

- 1/8 cup coconut oil

- 1/8 cup water

- 5 drops of peppermint oil

- 1/2 teaspoon on dried peppermint leaves

- 3 drops of rosemary oil

Use the hot process soap making method.

May 17

Lavender Fields and Chamomile Dreams Soap

- 1 lb. goat's milk soap

- 1/8 c. distilled water

- 2 T. Fine Ground Chamomile

- 2 T. Ground Lavender buds

- 1/8 c. Emu oil

- 5 drops lavender essential oil
- 2 drops roman chamomile essential oil

Use the hot process soap making method.

May 18

Sweet Baby Sudsy Soak

- 194 g lye
- 194 grams' lye
- 19 oz. water
- 8 oz. sweet almond oil
- 7 oz. jojoba
- 2 oz. castor oil
- 4 oz. shea butter
- 19 oz. coconut oil
- 14 oz. palm oil
- 1 oz. vitamin E oil

Use the cold process soap making method.

May 19

Herbal Milk Bath for Wee Ones

- 1 lb. Cornstarch
- 3 cups Goats Milk Powder
- 1/4 cup Lavender Powder

- 1/4 cup Calendula Petal Powder

- 1/2 cup Chamomile Powder

- 7 to 10 drops Lavender Essential Oil

- 2 drops Chamomile Essential Oil

Combine the lavender powder and lavender oil to a small bowl followed by the chamomile oil and powder. Then add in all of the remaining ingredients. Place herbal milk bath into a glass jar and use 1 tbsp. per baby size bath tub.

May 20

Cleansing Anti-Septic Tincture

- 1 tsp. goldenseal herb c/s

- 1/4 tsp. myrrh gum

- 1/4 tsp. calendula herb c/s

- 1 C. Everclear

Place the herbs in a glass jar and cover them with alcohol. Cap the jar and allow to sit for 2 weeks, shaking the jar each day. Strain the herbs and bottle.

May 21

Tea Rose Enchantment Bar Soap

- Castor Oil 2 oz.

- Coconut Oil 31 oz.

- Grapeseed Oil 20 oz.

- Olive Oil 21 oz.

- Palm Oil 8 oz.

- Safflower Oil 40 oz.

- Stearic Acid 3 oz.

- Lard 12 oz.
  Additives:

- 4 Oz. Castor Oil

- 1 Oz. Iron Oxide Colorant

- Â¼ Cup Aloe Vera Sap

- 1 Oz. Vitamin E

- Â¼ Cup Oatmeal Flour

- 4 Oz. Tea Rose Oil

- Lye Water

- 18 oz. Lye

- 4 Cups Distilled Water

Use the cold process soap making method.

May 22

Carrot Vegetable Soap Bar

Get your daily dose of veggies using this remarkable bar!

- 2 oz. sweet almond oil

- 4 oz. canola oil

- 8 oz. coconut oil

- 2 oz. palm kernel oil

- 8 oz. Hydrogenated Soybean oil

- 24 oz. total oils

- 1 Tbsp. Olive oil at trace for super fatting

- 1 Cup fresh Carrots

- 3.5 oz. lye

Use the cold process soap making method.

May 23

Lemon Olive Complexion Bar

- 2.6 oz. Sweet almond oil

- 2.6 oz. Castor oil

- 2.6 oz. Coconut oil

- 2.6 oz. Grapeseed oil

- 21.4 oz. Olive oil

- 4.3 oz. NaOH/Lye

- 11.4 fl oz. Water

- 1.4 oz. Lemongrass EO

Use the cold process soap making method.

May 24

Neem Oil Soap

- 18 oz. canola oil

- 18 oz. olive oil

- 5 oz. virgin coconut oil

- 4 oz. palm

- 4 oz. neem oil

- 2 oz. sesame oil

- 12 oz. of liquid

- 61/2 oz. of lye

- 1 T Tulsi

- 1 t Turmeric

- 1 t basil

- 1 t comfrey root

- 1 T neem powder

- 1 T Bentonite Clay

- 1 T Fullers Earth

- 1 T each of essential oil of Sandalwood & Myrrh

Use the cold process soap making method.

May 25

Vitalizing Vitamin Soap

- 3 lbs. (48 oz.) distilled water

- 475g Sodium Hydroxide

- 2-1/2 lbs. (40 oz.) Coconut Oil

- 1-1/2 lbs. (24 oz.) Palm Oil

- 1-3/4 lbs. (28 oz.) Olive Oil, Grade B or pomace (2 lbs less 1/2 cup)

- 1 oz. (2 tbsp.) Wheat Germ Oil

- 1 oz. (2 tbsp.) Carrot Seed Oil

- 1 oz. (2 tbsp.) Carrot Root Oil

- 1 oz. (2 tbsp.) Vitamin E Oi

- 1/2 lb. (8 oz.) Sweet Almond Oil

- 1/2 lb. (8 oz.) Apricot Kernel Oil

- 1/2 lb. (8 oz.) Kuku Nut Oil

- 1/2 lb. (8 oz.) Jojoba Oil

- 4 oz. Shea Butter

- 30g Grapefruit Seed Extract

- 2 oz. (4 tbsp.) Avocado Oil

- 2 oz. (4 tbsp.) Evening Primrose Oil, Borage Oil or Rosa Mosqueta Rosehip Seed Oil

- 45-50g (about 3 oz.) essential oils

Use the cold process soap making method.

May 26

English Countryside Soap

- 24 oz. Water

- 9 oz. Lye

- 20 oz. Coconut Oil

- 17.5 oz. Palm Oil

- 4.3oz Castor Oil

- 11.4 oz. Canola Oil

- 4.1 oz. Aloe Oil

- 5.1oz Sweet Almond Oil

- .8oz Shea Butter

- .8oz Cocoa Butter

- 1-1/2 tsp. Clove bud essential oil

- 1-1/2 tsp. Spearmint essential oil

- 1-1/2 tsp. Neroli fragrance oil

- 1/2 C. Calendula Petals at trace

Use the cold process soap making method.

May 27

Glowing Body Polish

- 2 oz. citrus blend or orange blossom floral water

- 1.5 oz. ground apricot kernel

- 1 oz. melt and pour glycerin soap

- 1 oz. aloe vera gel

- 1 oz. rice bran oil (or other light weight oil suitable for use on the face)

- Orange and Sandalwood essential oils

In a double boiler melt the soap. Once thoroughly melted, add the aloe vera gel and safflower oil. Remove from heat and stir in the floral water, a dropper of sandalwood oil and two droppers of orange essential oil. Mix thoroughly and then stir in the ground apricot kernel. Stirring frequently, allow the mixture to cool. Add more essential oil and floral water until the desired scent and consistency is achieved. Typically, the scrub is slightly more thin than creamy peanut butter. Scrape the scrub into glass containers and seal for a day or two. The ingredients will blend more thoroughly and fragrance will stabilize into a nutty, woody and vanilla scent.

Source:

https://www.fromnaturewithlove.com/recipe/recipe.asp?recipe_id=148

May 28

Vanilla Honey Oatmeal Bar

- 2lbs of clear or white melt and pour soap

- 1/8 to 1/4 cup of Honey

- 3/4 cup of ground oatmeal

- 1 tsp of vitamin E

- 1 tablespoon of Vanilla oil

- 1 tablespoon of Frankincense and Myrrh oil

Follow the melt and pour method.

May 29

Cucumber Ivy Mint Magic Soap Bar

- 1-pound opaque soap base

- 1 tablespoon cucumber fragrance oil

- 1 tablespoon English ivy fragrance oil

- 3-4 drops peppermint essential oil

- light green mica

Follow the melt and pour method.

May 30

Morning Coffee and Cream Sudz Bar

- 8 oz. Coconut Opaque melt and pour Base
- 2 tsp. Lanolin
- 2 tsp. Aloe Vera Gel
- 3 tsp. Coffee Grounds
- 2 tsp. Heavy Whipping Cream
- 10 Drops Coffee Fragrance Oil
- 10 Drops Vanilla Fragrance Oil

Follow the melt and pour method.

May 31

Super Sudsy Sea Sponge Soap

- 1 3-6-inch natural sea sponge
- 1 c. shea butter melt & pour soap
- 1 tbsp. buttermilk powder
- 1 tbsp. coconut milk powder
- 1 tbsp. lanolin
- Fragrance Oil of choice
- Powdered Mica of choice

Melt soap and lanolin and blend in powders completely. Add fragrance oil and mica. In large bowl, saturate sea sponge in soap while still quite warm and liquid. Remove sponge and drip off excess soap, let harden.

Source:

https://www.fromnaturewithlove.com/recipe/recipe.asp?recipe_id=486

June

Hello beautiful! Guess what? Summer is finally here! You've made it all the way through spring cleaning season. Now, it's time to sit back, relax, and enjoy the sunshine. During the month of June, we'll learn how to make more hot, cold, and melt and pour process soaps. Plan to stock up on all of your favorite scents and cute soap molds because it's going to be a soap-making extravaganza!

June 1

Calamine Lotion Soap Bar

Tell those itchy bug bites and heat rashes to take a hike with this fabulous soap bar made with soothing ingredients.

- 12 ounces of white glycerin or goats milk soap
- 2 tablespoons of calamine lotion
- 5 Vitamin E capsules
- 2 drops FDC Red #40
- 1/2 oz. bubblegum Fragrance oil

Follow the melt and pour method.

June 2

Choco Choco Crisp Soap Bar

This amazing soap bar is made with the scent of silky chocolate and is slightly textured for gentle exfoliation.

- 2 lb. Melt & Pour Soap Base

- 1/2 cup Goat's Milk Powder

- 1 tsp powdered Kola Nut (or other brown herb)

- 1 tsp Macadamia Nut Oil

- 1/2 tsp Cocoa Butter

- 1/2 tsp Mango Butter

- 1/2 tsp Silk Amino Acids

- Chocolate Fragrance Oil

Follow the melt and pour method.

June 3

Mega Citrus Sunshine Shampoo Bar

- 1 lb. opaque M&P base

- 1 tsp. almond oil

- 4 tsp. shea butter

- 1 ½ tsp. castor oil

- 1 oz. beeswax

- 1 ½ oz. cocoa butter

- 2-3 drops orange essential oil

- 2-3 drops lemon essential oil

- 2-3 drops grapefruit essential oil

Follow the melt and pour method.

June 4

Simple Coconut Vanilla Layer Soap Bar

- 2 oz. clear melt & pour base
- 2 oz. white melt & pour
- 10 drops chocolate fragrance
- 10 drops vanilla fragrance
- Cocoa powder or brown colorant

Follow the melt and pour method.

June 5

Berry Blast Smoothie Soap

- 1 lb. Shea Butter Melt and Pour Soap Base
- 1 to 2 tbsp. Blueberry Fibers
- 1 to 2 tbsp. Raspberry Fibers
- 3 tbsp. Goat's Milk Powder
- 1 tsp Virgin Coconut Oil
- 1 tsp Pistachio Butter
- 1/4 tsp Fragrance Oil

Follow the melt and pour method.

June 6

Sultry Hair Rinse

- 1 1/2 c. Distilled Water
- 2 tbsps. Haritaki Powder
- 2 tbsps. Hibiscus Petal Powder
- 1/2 c. Rosemary Hydrosol
- 1/2 c. Organic Apple Cider Vinegar

Bring ½ c. water to a boil and add the powdered herbs, stir. Reduce heat to low and simmer herbal liquid. Gentle boil for 30 minutes, covered. Remove mixture from heat and allow to cool. Once cooled, strain infusion through a cheesecloth into a pitcher. Add the ACV and rosemary hydrosol to the pitcher and stir. Add any optional scents at this time. Transfer hair rinse to flip top bottles.

June 7

Ginger Citrus Dry Shampoo

- 4 tbsps. white kaolin clay
- 2 tbsps. arrowroot powder
- 2 tbsps. powdered orange peel
- 2 drops Hawaiian white ginger fragrance oil
- 3 drops orange fragrance oil

Combine all dry ingredients followed by oils. Mix well and store in an airtight container.

June 8

Honey Almond Face Polish

- 1 tbsp. ground almonds
- 1 tbsp. colloidal oatmeal
- 1 tbsp. honey
- 1 tbsp. buttermilk powder
- Water

Mix all ingredients in a small mixing bowl, using enough water to create a thick paste. Smooth onto face using circular motions. Rinse with warm water and pat dry.

June 9

Gentleman's After Shave

After soapy up your skin and scraping away facial hair, you need to follow up with this amazing after shave.

- Distilled Water 11oz
- Aloe-Vera Gel 1:1 11oz
- Jojoba MP-44 8 oz.
- Fractionated Coconut oil 2oz
- Virgin Coconut Crème 3oz
- Wheat germ Oil .5oz
- Rice Bran Oil .5oz
- Kuku Nut Oil .5oz
- Carrot Oil .5oz
- Rosehip Seed Oil .5oz

- Borage Oil .5oz

- Hempseed Oil .5oz

- GSE 2ml

- Mango Butter 1.5oz

- Emulsifying Wax 1.8oz

- Fragrance of your choice

Place all ingredients into a microwave-safe bowl and heat to about 160 degrees. Once heated, use an immersion blender to mix concoction until smooth. Allow to sit on countertop until after shave cools to room temperature.

June 10

Milky Shea Butter Soap

- 8.6 ounces Canola Oil

- 8.6 ounces Coconut Oil

- 13.4 ounces Olive Oil

- 11.5 ounces Safflower Oil

- 5.8 ounces Shea Butter

- 47.0 ounces Vegetable Shortening

- 13.1 ounces Sodium Hydroxide (NaOH/Lye)

- 34.1 ounces Whole Milk

- 4.2 ounces Essential/Fragrance Oil

Follow Hot Process Soap Making Method.

June 11

Intense Moisture Bar

- 16.8 oz. Olive Oil (28%)
- 12 oz. Coconut Oil (20%)
- 9 oz. Palm Oil (15%)
- 7.2 oz. Emu Oil (12%)
- 3.6 oz. Castor Oil (6%)
- 3 oz. Avocado Oil (5%)
- 2.4 oz. Cocoa Butter (4%)
- 2.4 oz. Shea Butter (4%)
- 1.2 oz. Jojoba (2%)
- 1.2 oz. Sweet Almond Oil (2%)
- 23 oz. Distilled Water
- 8.14 oz. Lye (6% excess fat)
- Fragrance and color optional

Follow Hot Process Soap Making Method.

June 12

Peppermint Foot Scrub

- 4 oz. shea butter
- 4 oz. aloe butter
- 4 oz. fractionated coconut oil

- .75-1 cup dead sea salt (medium)
- .75-1 cup Epsom salt
- 1.5 teaspoon peppermint essential oil
- 1.5 teaspoon polysorbate 20

Using the double boiler method, melt shea butter to 170 degrees for 20 minutes. Remove from heat and allow to cool to about 130 degrees. Add the aloe butter, stirring until evenly mixed. Next, add the fractionated coconut oil. Allow mixture to cool to room temperature but don't allow to solidify. Mix in the essential oils and polysorbate 20. Add ¾ c. of each salt and stir. Transfer to jars and store in the refrigerator.

June 13

Summer-Inspired Salt Scrub

- 2 c. Sea Salt
- 1/2 c. Corn Meal
- 1/2 c. light oil
- 1 tsp. Soapnut or liquid soap (opt)
- Essential Oils like lemon, grapefruit, orange, and/or lime
- Powdered colorant

Place salt and cornmeal in a large bowl. Mix colorant and soapnut into the mixture. Add the essential oils and allow mixture to sit overnight, covered. Lastly, pour the oil and liquid soap into the mixture and stir. Transfer to a container and store in your shower for immediate use.

June 14

Perfectly Pear Soap Bar

- 6.4 oz. coconut oil

- 1.9 oz. illipe butter

- 4.8 oz. kokum butter

- 2.2 oz. lanolin

- 3.8 oz. mango butter

- 6.4 oz. palm kernel oil

- 3.2 oz. palm oil

- 3.2 oz. shea butter

- 11.5 oz. water

- 4.5 oz. lye

- Super fat with 1.1 oz. meadow foam oil and 1.1 oz. of avocado oil

- .7 oz. to 1.0 oz. pear berry fragrance

Follow the cold soap process soap making method.

June 15

Bubble Gum Kid-Approved Soap Bar

- 8 oz. soft water

- 3 oz. lye

- 7 oz. Crisco, palm oil or tallow

- 7 oz. coconut oil

- 6 oz. olive oil

- 1 oz. jojoba oil

- 1 oz. Bubble gum fragrance oil

- Imperial Red Mica to color

Follow the cold soap process soap making method.

June 16

Bug Repellant Soap

- 19.2 ounces' coconut oil

- 22.4 ounces olive Oil

- 16.0 ounces' palm Oil

- 6.4 ounces Shea Butter

- 6.4 ounces Neem Oil

- 23.0 ounces' water

- 9.6 ounces Sodium Hydroxide

- 14 teaspoons essential oil- equal parts Citronella Java, Eucalyptus Citriodora, Geranium and Rosemary essential oil

Follow the cold soap process soap making method.

June 17

Canola Oil Soap

- 4 oz. olive oil

- 52 oz. canola oil

- 9 oz. castor oil

- 30 oz. lard or tallow or Crisco or a combo, of any of them

- 28 oz. cold water

- 12 oz. lye

Follow the cold soap process soap making method.

June 18

Fabulous Flax Oil Soap

- 19.2 ounces Coconut oil

- 9.6 ounces Flax Seed oil

- 22.4 ounces Olive Oil

- 12.8 ounces Palm Oil

- 9.6 ounces Sodium Hydroxide

- 23 ounces' water

- 10 tsp. essential oil

Follow the cold soap process soap making method.

June 19

Precious Moments Soap

- 21.8 oz. Olive Oil

- 5.3 oz. Palm Oil

- 5.3 oz. Coconut Oil

- 4.3 oz. Lye

- 11.9 oz. Water

- 3 or 4 teaspoons fragrance oil

- 1 teaspoon herbal additives like ground chamomile

Follow the cold soap process soap making method.

June 20

Awesome Bar Soap Recipe

- 2.4 oz. Sweet Almond Oil

- 4.0 oz. Coconut Oil

- 3.4 oz. Grapeseed Oil

- 2.4 oz. Olive Oil

- 2.4 oz. Palm Oil

- 2.4 oz. Sunflower Oil

- Lye/Water:

- 2.4 oz. NaOH/Lye

- 5.7 oz. Water

Follow the cold soap process soap making method.

June 21

Honey Carrot Sweet Soap

- 13 oz. Fresh Carrot Juice

- 4.5 oz. Lye

- 16 oz. Vegetable Shortening

- 8 oz. Coconut Oil

- 4 oz. Cocoa Butter

- 4 oz. Sunflower Oil

- 2 Tbsp. Honey

- 2 Tbsp. Cucumber Fragrance Oil

- 1/4 tsp. Aloe Vera Fragrance Oil

Follow the cold soap process soap making method.

June 22

Lazy Day Summer Soap Recipe

- 5 1/2 oz. castor

- 30 oz. hydrogenated soy

- 40 oz. olive oil

- 16 oz. coconut oil

- 5 1/2 tsp each salt and sugar

- 12 1/2 oz. lye

- 34 oz. distilled water

Follow the cold soap process soap making method.

June 23

Pampering Soap Bar recipe

- 14.3 ounces' lye

- 34.5 ounces' water

- 2 tsp hydrolyzed silk amino acids added to water & lye mixture.

- 1.9 oz. sweet almond oil

- 19.2 oz. tallow (beef)
- 1.0 oz. castor oil
- 24.0 oz. coconut oil
- 1.0 oz. emu oil
- 1.9 oz. jojoba oil
- 1.9 oz. mango Butter
- 1.0 oz. neem oil
- 24.0 oz. olive oil
- 19.2 oz. palm oil
- 1.0 oz. sal butter
- 3 ounces of mango butter, 2 ounces of jojoba oil, and 2 ounces of emu oi

Follow the cold soap process soap making method.

June 24

Peppermint Perk Soap Bar

- 1 tbsp. Peppermint essential oil
- 1 tsp. Rosemary essential oil
- 1 tsp. Tea Tree essential oil
- .25 grams T50 or ROE
- 1/3 cup peppermint leaves, finely ground

Follow the cold soap process soap making method.

June 25

Big, Beautiful Bubbles Soap Bar

- 8 oz. sweet almond oil

- 2 oz. castor oil

- 10 oz. coconut oil

- 10 oz. olive oil

- 8 oz. safflower oil

- 10 oz. vegetable shortening

- 7 oz. lye (5% super fat)

- 17 oz. water

Follow the cold soap process soap making method.

June 26

Tantalizing Tea Bar

- 8 oz. fractionated coconut oil

- 8 oz. soybean oil

- 8 oz. olive oil

- 4 oz. aloe butter

- 4 oz. shea butter

- 4 oz. butter (unsalted)

- 3 tea bags - chamomile or green tea

- 1 tsp chamomile essential oil

- 1/2 cup chopped cucumber

- 12 oz. water

- 5.2 oz. lye

Follow the cold soap process soap making method.

June 27

Mother Earth Soap

- 1 lb. unscented clear glycerin melt & pour base

- 1 1/2tsp. ground cinnamon, divided

- 10 drops sweet orange essential oil

- 5 drops lavender essential oil

- 1 drop rosemary essential oil

- 1 tsp. sunflower oil

Follow melt and pour soap process method.

June 28

Fancy English-Inspired Soap

- 1 lb. Avocado & Cucumber glycerin soap base, cubed

- 1 Tablespoon avocado butter

- 2 oz. cucumber

- 1/2 teaspoon lemon juice

- 1 chamomile tea bag (opened)

- 30 drops Roman Chamomile essential oil

Follow melt and pour soap process method.

June 29

French Citrus Soap Bar

- 8 oz. melt and pour (clear or opaque)
- 1 tsp French Green Clay
- 1/2 tsp. Lemon Peel Powder
- 1/2 tsp. Orange Peel Powder
- 1 tsp. Jojoba Oil
- 5 drops Tea Tree Essential Oil
- 5 drops Lemon Essential Oil
- 2 drops Lemongrass Essential Oil

Follow melt and pour soap process method.

June 30

Honey Bee Baby Soap

- 4 oz. honey melt and pour soap
- 1 tbsp. beeswax
- 1 tbsp. honey
- Pinch of bee pollen

Follow melt and pour soap process method.

July

Summer is now officially in full swing! How are you enjoying your soap making adventures? I bet you have quite a stockpile of fresh and fun soaps, don't you? During the month of July, when the sun is in full force, we'll focus on taking good care of our skin. From soothing soaps for sun burn to gentle facial scrubs, July has got your fun-in-the-sun needs covered.

July 1

Skin Loving Soap Bar

- 1 lb. any opaque melt and pour soap base
- 4 tsp. Green Clay powder
- 12 drops eucalyptus essential oil
- Pinch of chromium oxide green if desired

Follow melt and pour soap process method.

July 2

Glorious Lemon Rosemary Soap Bar

When you've been chopping up garlic and onions to throw on the BBQ, this skin-loving soap will help combat those odors from your hands.

- 2 lbs. clear melt and pour base
- Lemon essential oil
- Lime essential oil
- 4 tsp. dried rosemary leaves

Follow melt and pour soap process method.

July 3

Love Your Body Soap

- 8 oz. shea or cocoa butter melt and pour soap base
- 2 tbsps. shea butter
- 1 tbsp. cocoa butter
- 2 tbsps. finely ground oatmeal 1 tbsp. rose petal powder
- 20 drops red colorant
- 40 drops rose geranium essential oil
- 20 drops ylang-ylang essential oil

Follow melt and pour soap process method.

July 4

Butter Lover's Bodacious Bod Soap

Suds up with this soap after a day at the beach.

- 1 lb. Melt & Pour Soap Base (any)
- 1/4 tsp. Emu Oil, Grade A
- 1/4 tsp. Vitamin E Oil, 1000 IU
- 1 1/2 tsp. Cocoa Butter
- 1 1/2 tsp. Mango Butter
- Fragrance or essential oil of choice

Follow melt and pour soap process method.

July 5

Love Your Face Bar

- 1 lb. rosehip and jojoba melt and pour base

- 2 tsp. French green or Moroccan red clay

- 1/2 tsp. of avocado oil

- 1/2 tsp. of apricot or peach kernel oil

- 1/2-ounce fragrance or essential oil

Follow melt and pour soap process method.

July 6

Leftover Soap Madness!

- 1 to 3 different colored soaps – Left Overs work best!

- Clear base

- White base

- 2" tube mold

- 1/2" tube mold or dowel

Follow melt and pour soap process method.

July 7

Milk and Honey Baby Bar

- 2 Tablespoons Olive Oil

- 2 Tablespoons Water
- 2 Tablespoons Milk Powder
- 2 Tablespoons Honey, natural not powdered
- Honey, Spice or Vanilla Fragrance Oil
- 1/2 cup melted Melt and Pour base

Follow melt and pour soap process method.

July 8

One with Nature Soap

- 1 lb. any melt and pour soap base
- 1/4 cup clay of choice
- 2 tbsp. lanolin
- 1 tbsp. high oleic sunflower seed oil
- 1 tbsp. vitamin E, 1000 IU oil
- 4 drops mandarin essential oil
- 3 drops Spanish lemon essential oil

Follow melt and pour soap process method.

July 9

Herbal Soap Scrolls

- 8 oz. clear melt & pour base
- 1/4 cup herbs
- Fragrance oil

Follow melt and pour soap process method. During last phase, while soap is still warm, roll into "scrolls" and secure with raffia.

July 10

Orange Mocha Garden Bars

- 1 lb. opaque melt and pour soap

- 3 tbsp. food grade cocoa butter

- 1 tbsp. coconut oil

- 1/4 c. finely ground coffee

- 1 tbsp. fragrance oil blend

- Cocoa powder or umber oxide to color the mixture a light creamed coffee color

Orange Mocha Dream Fragrance Oil Recipe:

- 1 tbsp. orange essential oil

- 1 1/2 tsp cappuccino or coffee fragrance oil

- 1/2 tsp chocolate fragrance oil

Follow melt and pour soap process method.

July 11

Get Relaxed Soap Bar

- 1 lb. M&P goats milk soap

- 2 tsp. Beeswax

- 1 tbsp. Solid Coconut Oil

- 2 tbsp. powdered green tea

- 2 tbsp. lavender powder

- 1/2 tsp. lavender fragrance oil

- 1/4 tsp. cucumber fragrance oil

- 1/4 tsp. bergamot fragrance oil

- 5 drops green tea fragrance oil

- Green and purple colorant

Follow melt and pour soap process method.

July 12

Soap for My Summertime Lover

- 1 oz. heart shaped chocolate mold

- 4 oz. round soap mold

- 1 oz. MP soap (clear or white)

- 3 drops clove oil

- 2 drops cinnamon oil

- 2 drops buttercream fragrance

- FDC dye for deep red or burgundy coloring

- 3 oz. clear melt and pour soap

- 2 drops buttercream fragrance

Follow melt and pour soap process method.

July 13

Rosy Complexion Bar

- 4 oz. melt and pour soap base

- 10 drops rose essential oil

- 5 drops Tea Tree oil

- 1/2 tsp. Jojoba oil

- Red color

Follow melt and pour soap process method.

July 14

Oceania Soap

- 1 lb. suspension melt & pour base

- 2 tbsps. Kelp powder

- 2 tbsps. flax seed meal

- 15-20 drops Tea Tree essential oil

Follow melt and pour soap process method.

July 15

Exfoliating Honey Oatmeal Bath Bar

- 2 lbs. of clear or white melt and pour soap

- 1/8 to 1/4 cup of Honey

- 3/4 c. of ground oatmeal

- 1 tsp. of vitamin E

- 1 tbsp. of Vanilla oil

- 1 tbsp. of Frankincense and Myrrh essential oil

Follow melt and pour soap process method.

July 16

Azuki Bean Cucumber Kokum Skin Nourishing Soap Bar

- Freshly grounded Azuki Beans [you can get these in Asian stores] 1/2 cup
- 4 oz. of Cucumber Floral Water
- 4 oz. of Neroli Hydrosol
- 3 oz. castor oil
- 6 oz. coconut oil
- 2 oz. Kokum butter
- 4 oz. olive oil
- 4 oz. palm oil
- 1 oz. Sunflower oil
- 2.83 oz.lye [NaOH]
- Mandarin Orange essential oil
- Basil Fragrance oil
- Sprinkle of chamomile leaves
- Vitamin E T50
- Green mica

Follow cold process soap making method.

July 17

Boozy Bay Rum Soap Bar

- Tallow (beef) 10 oz.

- Sesame seed oil (untoasted) 6 oz.

- Olive oil 6 oz.

- Coconut oil 6 oz.

- Palm kernel flakes 6 oz.

- Castor oil 2 oz.

- Rice bran oil 1 oz.

- Lye (at 5% discount) 5.28 oz.

- Water 14 oz. OR 12.6 oz. (discounted)

- .5 to 1 oz. Bay Rum fragrance oil

Follow cold process soap making method.

July 18

Super Sweet Honey Almond Body Bar

- 1 oz. Beeswax

- 8.6 oz. Coconut Oil

- 3.2 oz. Olive Oil

- 19.2 oz. Soybean Oil

- 4.8 oz. Lye

- 9.6 oz. Water

- 1 tsp. Salt

- 0.5 oz. Almond fragrance oil

- 0.5 oz. Honey fragrance oil

Follow cold process soap making method.

July 19

Exfoliating Milk and Honey Bee Soap

- 4 oz. beeswax

- 5 oz. sweet almond oil

- 15 oz. coconut oil

- 15 oz. palm oil

- 25 oz. vegetable shortening

- 8.7 oz. lye

- 24 oz. water/milk or water and milk mixture

- 1 oz. honey

- Cinnamon powder for sprinkling at trace

- 1/2 cups colloidal oatmeal coarse

- Oatmeal, Milk and Honey fragrance oil

Follow cold process soap making method.

July 20

All About Milk Based Soap

- 1 cup vegetable shortening

- 1/2 cup melted coconut oil

- 1/2 cup palm oil

- 1 cup milk, cream, or powdered milk

- 1/4 cup Red Devil lye granules

- 1/4 cup water

- 1 1/2 teaspoons essential oil

Follow cold process soap making method.

July 21

Minty Chocolate Soap

- 8 oz. Palm Oil

- 7 oz. Coconut Oil

- 10.5 oz. Olive Oil

- 10.5 oz. Canola Oil

- 3 oz. Cocoa Butter

- 16 oz. Water

- 6 oz. Lye

- Peppermint fragrance oil

- 2 tbsps. Cocoa Powder

- 2 tbsps. Castor Oil

Follow cold process soap making method.

July 22

Grandpa's Old-Fashioned Goat's Milk Soap

- 12 oz. lard

- 1.5 lbs. coconut oil

- 1.5 lbs. avocado oil

- 11 oz. water
- 10 oz. lye
- 10 oz. goats milk
- 1 tablespoon dill weed-finely chopped
- 1 tablespoon anise essential oil
- 3 tablespoons fennel essential oil
- 1 1/2 teaspoons grapefruit seed extract

Follow cold process soap making method.

July 23

Silky Smooth Shampoo Bar

- Sweet Almond Oil 8 oz.
- Canola Oil 8 oz.
- Castor Oil 24 oz.
- Coconut Oil 32 oz.
- Olive Oil 32 oz.
- Palm Oil 24 oz.
- Lye 17.95 oz.
- Liquid 46 oz.
- Essential oil to scent

Follow cold process soap making method.

July 24

Sweet Summer Rays Soap Bar

- 15 oz. canola oil

- 30 oz. Coconut oil

- 27 oz. Olive oil

- 21 oz. Palm oil

- 5 oz. Shea butter

- 13.75 oz. Lye

- 20 oz. Rain or distilled water

- 16 oz. pureed cucumber

Follow cold process soap making method.

July 25

Simply Shea Butter Soap

- 4.8 oz. olive oil

- 4.8 oz. coconut oil

- 3.2 oz. shea butter

- 3.2 oz. palm oil

- 6oz distilled water

- 2.2oz of lye

- .8oz essential oil

Follow cold process soap making method.

July 26

Sow Your Wild Oats Soap Bar

- 1 oz. cocoa butter

- 11 oz. coconut oil

- 16 oz. olive oil

- 4 oz. beeswax

- 4.32 oz. lye

- 12 oz. water

- 4 oz. course colloidal oatmeal

Follow cold process soap making method.

July 27

White Zinfandel Soap

- Tallow (beef) 6 oz.

- Olive oil 4 oz.

- Coconut oil 3 oz.

- Grapeseed oil 2 oz.

- Castor oil 1 oz.

- Lye (discount at 6%) 2.19 oz.

- 6 oz. chilled precooked wine

- .5 oz. Wine fragrance oil

- Light rose or pink colorant

Follow cold process soap making method. Cook wine until boiling so
that it may release its alcohol.

July 28

Sunny Complexion Soap Bar

- 1.6 oz. Sweet Almond Oil

- 0.6 oz. Cocoa Butter

- 9.6 oz. Olive Oil

- 8.0 oz. Palm Kernel Oil

- 12.2 oz. Shortening (veg)4.5 oz. Sodium Hydroxide (NaOH/Lye)

- 11.5 oz. Water

- 1.4 oz. total of Essential/Fragrance Oil

- Essential Oil: Roman Chamomile; .2 oz.

- Essential Oil: Rose Bulgarian; .2 oz.

- Essential Oil: Lavender; 1 oz.

- Dried Herbs: 1 oz. total: Rose Powder, Chamomile powder and Calendula powder

Follow cold process soap making method.

July 29

Dead Sea Rejuvenating Face Mask

- 1/2 cup Dead Sea Mud

- 4 drops Lavender Essential Oil

- 3 drops German Chamomile Essential Oil

- 1 drop Peppermint Essential Oil

Blend mud carefully with essential oils, mixing completely and store in an airtight container.

July 30

Enchanted Beauty Facial Love

- 1 tsp. Rose Clay
- 1 egg white
- 1/16th tsp. Neem Powder
- 1/2 tsp. oat starch
- Rose hydrosol

Mix all ingredients but the rose hydrosol carefully together. Once mixed, slowly add the rose hydrosol until desired consistency is reached. Apply to face and allow to sit for 15 minutes. Wash off with a mild soap and warm water. Pat skin dry.

July 31

Mango Mint Shampoo Bar

- 1 cup grated soap
- 1/2 cup water
- 1/4 cup olive oil
- 1/4 cup castor oil
- 1 t dried crushed peppermint leaves
- 15 drops mango fragrance oil

Follow hot process soap making method.

August

Wow! Hasn't the summer been moving quickly? Here, we find ourselves already in August. Summer is almost at an end, but we still have lots of soap making to do. August focuses on all things bath time. Are you ready to continue on this sudsy adventure? Great! Let's keep going.

August 1

Two Lovers Aphrodisiac Bath Oil

- ½ oz. Rose fragrance oil
- 1/8 oz. Ylang ylang fragrance oil
- ¼ oz. Sandalwood fragrance oil
- 1/16 oz. Patchouli fragrance oil
- 1/16 oz. Neroli fragrance oil
- 1 oz. Amber Glass Bottle with dropper

Mix all ingredients into an amber glass bottle, cap, and shake.

August 2

Cleansing Bath Salts

- 1 c. pink Himalayan salt
- 1 c. almond oil

Mix ingredients together and store in a glass jar.

August 3

Fizzy Bath Bombs

- 1/2 cup baking soda

- 1/4 cup citric acid

- 1/4 cup cornstarch

- 4 teaspoons sunflower oil

- 1 teaspoon water

- 1 teaspoon fragrance oil or essential oil

- 1/8 teaspoon borax

Mix the first 3 ingredients together in a mixing bowl. In another bowl, combine oil, water, fragrance, and borax followed by any colorant you plan to use. Pour both bowls of ingredients into a large jar, cap, and shake. Next, press concoction into molds and allow to dry overnight. Remove bath bombs and use.

August 4

Soapy Bath Syrup

- 2 cups of vegetable glycerin

- 1 cup of bubble bath

- 1/3 cup of turkey red oil

- 1 tablespoon of vanilla bean fragrance oil

- 1 tablespoon of freshly brewed coffee fragrance oil

Combine all ingredients into a dark bottle, cap, and shake. Use 3 tbsps. per tub.

August 5

Little Girl's Pink Bath Fairy Dust

- 1 Cup Epsom Salt
- 1 Cup Bolivian Pink Salt, Fine
- 1/2 Teaspoon Silver Sparkle Mica
- 2 Drops Bergamot Essential Oil
- 2 Drops Geranium Essential Oil
- 1 Drop Rose Absolute or 2 Drops Rose Essential Oil

Combine all ingredients into a mixing bowl and stir. Store in a glass jar. Use 2-4 tbsps. per bath.

August 6

Little Boys' Blue Bath Gnome Dust

- 1 Cup Epsom Salt
- 1 Cup Dead Sea Salt, Fine
- 1/2 Teaspoon Cobalt Mica
- 1 Teaspoon Silver Sparkle Mica
- 5-6 Drops Lavender Essential Oil

Combine all ingredients into a mixing bowl and stir. Store in a glass jar. Use 2-4 tbsps. per bath.

August 7

Chocolate Bath Cream

- 1 cup of powdered chocolate
- 1 cup of cocoa butter
- 1 cup of apricot kernel oil
- 1/2 cup of grapeseed oil
- 1 cup of cocoa butter melt and pour soap
- 1 teaspoon of warm vanilla sugar fragrance oil

Heat the cocoa butter over a double boiler until melted, then add the oils. Using an immersion blender, mix the concoction well. During the blending phase, drizzle the melt and pour soap base and fragrance oil into the solution. Place the bath cream into jars and allow to cool overnight. Add 1-2 tbsps. under running water.

August 8

End of Summer Chocolate Bath Fizzers

- 1/4 cup citric acid
- 1/4 cup corn starch
- 2 tbsp. cocoa powder
- 7 tbsp. coconut oil melted

Mix dry ingredients. Then, melt coconut oil and slowly drizzle over dry ingredients. Stir together well. Use an ice cream scoop to make 3 scoops and unmold them onto waxed paper and allow to dry for 48-hours.

August 9

Pretty Skin Flower Bath Salts

- 1 cup of your preferred salts relatively coarse salts: Epsom, sea salt, Dead Sea salts, etc.

- 3 tsp. dendritic salt

- 2 tsp. borax

- 1 - 2 tsp. liquid glycerin

- 12 drops alkanet-infused almond oil or infuse it in any other non-greasy oil by heating them up in a double boiler and straining through a tea bag or coffee filter

- 1/8 tsp jojoba oil

- 15 drops ylang ylang essential oil

- 10 drops lavender essential oil

Mix the first 3 ingredients together in a mixing bowl. In another bowl, combine glycerin, oil, fragrance, and borax followed by any colorant you plan to use. Pour both bowls of ingredients into a large jar, cap, and shake. Next, press concoction into molds and allow to dry overnight. Remove bath bombs and use.

August 10

Flower Child Herbal Hippie Soak

- 1 cup patchouli leaves

- 1/4 cup blue lavender buds

- 1 handful chamomile flowers

- 1 handful calendula petals

- 5 drops amber fragrance

Place all herbs into an airtight container and allow to sit overnight. Place 4 tbsps. in a muslin sachet and add to hot bath water.

August 11

Honey Body Wash

- 1 tbsp. Dead Sea clay

- 1 tsp. of yucca root powder

- 2 tbsp. of organic flaxseed oil

- 2 cups liquid castile

- 10 drops of your favorite essential oil

Place Dead Sea clay, yucca root, and flaxseed oil into a blender and pulse until smooth. Next, add 1 ½ cups of castile soap to the mixture and blend some more. Pour mixture into a bottle or jar and use with a loofah or sponge.

August 12

Tub Tea

- 1 cup powdered milk

- 1 cup colloidal oatmeal

- 1 cup wheat bran

- 1 cup lavender buds

- 10 drops lavender essential oil

- 5 large heat sealable tea bags

Mix all dry ingredients in a large bowl followed by the lavender oil. Scoop into teabags and seal. Add one teabag per filled tub.

August 13

End of Summer Bath Soak

- 9 drops Bergamot essential oil

- 10 drops Nutmeg essential oil

- 6 drops Clary Sage essential oil

Combine this woodsy blend with your favorite carrier oil and drip a few drops into your bath water.

August 14

Bath Candy

- 4 oz. cocoa butter

- 1 oz. colloidal oatmeal / fine

- 4 oz. grapeseed oil

- 10 drops of butter cream fragrance oil

Combine cocoa butter and grapeseed oil in a bowl and melt then add oatmeal and fragrance oils and mix very well. Pour into greased tart containers.

Source:

https://www.fromnaturewithlove.com/recipe/recipe.asp?recipe_id=531

August 15

Silky Bath Soak

- 1-part sunflower seeds
- 1-part corn starch
- 2-parts finely ground oats
- 2-parts milk powder
- Fragrance

Coarsely grind seeds in a blender or food processor. Add remaining ingredients and mix. Now, add your choice of fragrance oil. Store in a glass jar and add as much as you want to your bath water.

August 16

Raspberry Passion Sugar Scrub

- 6 oz. Turbinado Sugar
- 4 oz. Coconut oil
- 2 oz. Shea Butter
- 2 oz. Virgin Olive Oil
- 2 oz. Dendritic Salt
- 1 tbsp. Raspberry Fruit Fiber
- 1 tbsp. Black Raspberry Seeds
- 10 drops Clary Sage Essential Oil
- 8 drops Patchouli Essential Oil

- 6 drops Sandalwood Essential Oil

- 4 drops Ylang Ylang Essential Oil

- 8 drops Vitamin E (T-50)

Warm oils just until melted in the microwave or double boiler. In another bowl, place the dendritic salt, essential oils, and vitamin E. Blend together. Add in the raspberry fruit fiber and black raspberry seeds to the salt mixture. Add the oil solution to the dry mixture and stir. Store in an airtight container.

August 17

White Chocolate and strawberry Sugar Scrub

- 1 cup demerara or turbinado sugar

- 2 oz. cocoa butter

- 1 oz. strawberry seed oil

- 1 tbsp. strawberry seeds

- 20 drops strawberry fragrance oil

Melt the cocoa butter, and add the strawberry oil. Mix all dry ingredients together and stir well. Pour oil mixture over dry mixture and stir. Add scrub to an airtight container.

August 18

Hygienic Body Powder

- 1/3 cup cornstarch

- 1/3 cup arrowroot powder

- 1/3 cup oatmeal fine
- ¼ tsp. Mica
- Essential Oil

Mix all ingredients together and store in a glass shaker jar.

August 19

Hot Weather Cooling Foot Powder

Not only does this powder cool your angry dogs, it also keeps them fresh and stink-free.

- 1 tsp. finely ground peppermint
- ¼ c. cornstarch
- ¾ c. baking soda
- 1 tsp. white clay
- 25-30 drops peppermint and spearmint essential oils

Mix all ingredients together in a small bowl and transfer to a glass jar. Shake well before each use.

August 20

Summer Soap Jellies

- 9 Cube Soap Silicone Mold
- 32 oz. Stephenson Jelly Melt and Pour
- 10 mL Summer Fling Fragrance Oil
- 1/2 tsp. Fine Iridescent Glitter
- Fuchsia Lab Color

- Canary LabColor

- Orange LabColor

- Optional: Droppers

Follow the melt and pour soap making method.

August 21

Lemony Goat's Milk Soap Bars

- Goat Milk Tray Mold

- 28 oz. Goat Milk Melt and Pour Base

- 10 mL Lemon Essential Oil

- 1.5 tsp. Lemon Peel

- Yellow Oxide Color Block

Follow the melt and pour soap making method.

August 22

Kids' Bath Crayons

- 4 oz. clear melt and pour block

- 18 Lip Balm Tubes

- Lip Balm Pouring Tray (optional)

- 3 mL White Tea and Ginger Fragrance Oil

- Red LabColor (small)

- Orange LabColor (small)

- Canary LabColor (small)

- Emerald LabColor (small)
- Brilliant Blue LabColor (small)

ONE: In a heat-safe container, cut and melt the clear melt and pour soap in the microwave. Melt the soap in 10 second bursts, stirring in between each burst. Next, add 3 mL of White Tea and Ginger Fragrance Oil. Stir well. If you are using the Lip Balm Pouring Tray, put the lip balm tubes into the tray. The tray makes it easy to pour the soap into the tubes!

TWO: Pour .6 oz. of the melted clear soap in a small container. Then, and add 1 mL of the undiluted Red LabColor and use a spoon to incorporate. If need be, melt the soap in the microwave using 2 second bursts. That makes it easier to pour. Pour the melted soap into three of the lip balm tubes and spray with 99% isopropyl alcohol to pop any bubbles.

THREE: Pour .6 oz. of melted soap in a small container, and then add 1 mL of undiluted Orange LabColor. Mix the color in well. If need be, melt the soap in the microwave using 2 second bursts. That makes it easier to pour. Pour the soap into three of the lip balm tubes and spray with 99% isopropyl alcohol to pop any bubbles.

FOUR: Repeat this process with the green, yellow and blue colors. If need be, melt the soap in the microwave using 2 second bursts. That makes it easier to pour.

FIVE: For the purple color, we found the best results came from a mix of Red LabColor with Brilliant Blue LabColor. To get the color, we mixed 7 drops Red LabColor with 3 drops Brilliant Blue LabColor.

Stir to incorporate the colors, and pour the soap into three lip balm tubes.

SIX: Let the soap fully cool and harden for about 30 minutes. Remove the tubes from the tray and enjoy!

Source: http://teachsoap.com/2015/04/08/melt-and-pour-bath-crayons/

August 23

Cherry Soda Cupcake Cuties

- 16 oz. White Melt & Pour Base
- Cupcake Mold
- 1/2 oz. Cherry Pop Fragrance Oil
- Bright Cherry LabColor
- Canary Labcolor

Follow the melt and pour soap making method.

August 24

Succulent tangerine Soap

- 16 oz. shea melt and pour soap base
- 1 tsp. tangerine essential oil
- ½ tsp. 10x orange essential oil
- ¼ tsp. spearmint essential oil
- ¼ tsp. yellow oxide

Follow the melt and pour soap making method.

August 24

Vanilla Bean Oatmeal Bar

- 2lbs of clear or white melt and pour soap
- 3/4 cup of ground oatmeal
- 1 tsp of vitamin E
- 1 tablespoon of Vanilla Bean fragrance oil

Follow the melt and pour method.

August 25

Vanilla Rose Soap Bar

- 2lbs of clear or white melt and pour soap
- 3/4 cup of ground oatmeal
- 1 tsp of vitamin E
- 1 tablespoon of Vanilla oil
- 1 tablespoon of Rose oil

Follow the melt and pour method.

August 26

Honey Lemon Tea Bar

- 2lbs of clear or white melt and pour soap
- 1/8 to 1/4 cup of Honey
- 3/4 cup of ground black tea
- 1 tsp of vitamin E

- 1 tablespoon of vanilla essential oil
- 1 teaspoon of lemon essential oil

Follow the melt and pour method.

August 27

Floral Bouquet Bars

- 2lbs of clear or white melt and pour soap
- 3/4 cup of ground lilac, rose, and lavender petals
- 1 tsp of vitamin E
- 1 tablespoon of floral fragrance oil

Follow the melt and pour method.

August 28

Red Rooibos Tea Bar

- 2lbs of clear or white melt and pour soap
- 1/8 to 1/4 cup of Honey
- 3/4 cup of ground red rooibos tea
- 1 tsp of vitamin E
- 1 tablespoon of vanilla essential oil
- 1 teaspoon of lemon essential oil

Follow the melt and pour method.

August 29

Baby Powder Scent Bar

- 2lbs of clear or white melt and pour soap
- 1 tsp of vitamin E
- 1 tablespoon of Baby Powder fragrance oil

Follow the melt and pour method.

August 30

Honey Suckle Soap Bar

- 2lbs of clear or white melt and pour soap
- 1/8 to 1/4 cup of Honey
- 1 tsp of vitamin E
- 1 tablespoon of honey suckle fragrance oil
- 1 teaspoon of jasmine essential oil

Follow the melt and pour method.

August 31

Honey Olive Bar

- 2lbs of clear or white melt and pour soap
- 1/8 to 1/4 cup of Honey
- ½ cup olive oil
- 1 tsp of vitamin E
- 1 tablespoon of olive fragrance oil

Follow the melt and pour method.

September

Summer is over and it's time to get back to basics. School is in session, people are going back to work, and vacations are over. Whatever shall you do? Make soap! This section of the book will focus on creating soaps for the impending cooler months of fall. It might be time to put the sunscreen and flip flops away, but keep out your soap making supplies.

September 1

Apricot Yum Yum Soap

- 163 grams Shea Butter
- 163 grams Mango Butter
- 340 grams Apricot Kernel Oil
- 299 grams Avocado Oil
- 395 grams Coconut Oil 76
- 84 grams Apricot Fragrance Oil

Follow the hot process soap making method.

September 2

Argan Oil Soap

- 172 grams of water
- 64 grams of Lye
- 77 grams of Avocado Oil

144

- 136 grams of Coconut Oil 76

- 68 grams of Argan Oil

- 100 grams of Mango Butter

- 73 grams of Sunflower Oil

- 28 grams of Kulu Bay Fragrance Oil

- 25 grams of Sodium Lactate

- 20 grams of Vanilla White Color Stabilizer

Follow the hot process soap making method.

September 3

Awapuhi Sea Berry Soap

- 517 grams of water

- 189 grams of lye

- 272 grams of Olive Oil pomace

- 272 grams of Shea Butter

- 354 grams of Coconut Oil 76

- 136 grams of Cocoa Butter

- 231 grams of Sweet Almond Oil

- 95 grams of Castor Oil

- 85 grams of Awapuhi Seaberry Fragrance Oil

- 60 grams of Sodium Lactate

Follow the hot process soap making method.

September 4

Adorable Baby Shower Gift Soap

- 517 grams of water
- 195 grams of Lye
- 272 grams of Cocoa Butter
- 408 grams of Palm Oil
- 204 grams of Fractionated Coconut Oil
- 204 grams of Olive Oil Pomace
- 272 grams of Shea Butter
- 85 grams of New Born Baby Fragrance Oil

Follow the hot process soap making method.

September 5

Bastille Soap

- 12.16 oz Water (345 grams)
- 4.4 oz Lye (NaOH) (125 grams)
- 24 oz Olive Oil (680 grams)
- 6.4 oz Coconut Oil (181.5 grams)
- 1.6 oz Castor Oil (45.4 grams)
- Fun Liquid Soap Dyes (optional)
- 1.5 oz. Drakkar Type Fragrance Oil

Follow the hot process soap making method.

September 6

Brewsky Bar Soap

- Beer
- 517 grams Beer
- 186 grams Lye
- 408 grams Olive Oil Pomace
- 408 grams Shea Butter
- 272 grams Coconut Oil 76
- 272 grams Palm Oil
- 84 grams STUD Fragrance Oil

Follow the hot process soap making method.

September 7

Blackberry Sage Soap

- 150 grams- Diamond Clear Melt and Pour Soap Base
- 6 grams- Blackberry Sage Fragrance Oil
- 9 drops Fun Soap Colorant Ultramarine Violet
- 1 drop Fun Soap Colorant Black Oxide

Follow the melt and pour making method.

September 8

Scrumptious Blueberry Cheesecake Soap Bars

- 259 grams Water
- 258 grams 2% Milk
- 196 grams Lye
- 449 grams Palm Oil
- 191 grams Coconut Oil 76
- 163 grams Olive Oil Pomace
- 218 grams Shea Butter
- 136 grams Castor Oil
- 68 grams Safflower Oil
- 136 grams Fractionated Coconut Oil
- 84 grams Vanilla White Color Stabilizer
- 84 grams Blueberry Cheesecake Fragrance Oil
- 4 grams Titanium Dioxide
- 36 drops Ultramarine Blue Fun Soap Colorant
- 4 drops Deep Purple Fun Soap Colorant
- 1 drop Black Oxide Soap Colorant

Follow the cold process soap making method.

September 9

Warm and Sunny Calendula Soap

- Water: 197 grams

- Aloe Vera Juice: 98 grams

- Lye: 126 grams11 oz Olive Oil (312 grams)

- 10.5 oz Coconut Oil (297.6 grams)

- 7 oz Rice Bran Oil (198.5 grams)

- 1.5 oz Shea Butter (42.5 grams)

- 1.5 oz Mango butter (42.5 grams)

- 2 oz. Breezes and Sunshine Fragrance Oil

Follow the cold process soap making method.

September 10

Creamy Calendula Swirl Soap Bar

- 517 grams Distilled Water

- 194 grams Lye

- 408 Olive Oil- Pomace

- 408 Coconut Oil 76

- 408 Palm Oil

- 68 grams Castor Oil

- 68 grams Grapeseed Oil

- 90 grams Aromatherapy Energizing Fragrance

- 55 grams Sodium Lactate

- 3 grams Orange Oxide

- 3 grams Neon Yellow

- 1 grams Yellow Oxide

- 20 grams Titanium Dioxide

Follow the hot process soap making method.

September 11

Carmel and Custard Creamy Soap

- 259 grams Water
- 258 grams Evaporated Milk
- 188 grams Lye
- 340 grams Palm Oil
- 340 grams Coconut Oil 76
- 408 grams Shea Butter
- 204 grams Grapeseed Oil
- 68 grams Castor Oil
- 84 grams Vanilla White Color Stabilizer (added to the fragrance oil)
- 84 grams Caramel Custard Fragrance Oil
- 2 grams Titanium Dioxide

Follow the cold process soap making method.

September 12

Bunny Bliss Carrot Soap

- 8.5 oz Water (241 grams)
- 4.5 oz Lye (127.5 grams)
- 4 oz Carrot Baby Food (add at the same time as the lye water and bring to trace) (113 grams)
- 15 oz Olive Oil (425 grams)

- 8 oz Coconut Oil (227 grams)

- 4 oz Castor Oil (113 grams)

- 3 oz Cocoa Butter (85 grams)

- 3 oz Shea Butter (85 grams)

- 2 oz. Frosted Pumpkin Fragrance Oil

Follow the cold process soap making method.

September 13

Classic Cleo Heavy Cream Soap

- 387 grams Water

- 130 grams Frozen Heavy Whipping Cream

- 196 grams Lye

- 449 grams Palm Oil

- 191 grams Coconut Oil 76

- 163 grams Olive Oil Pomace

- 218 grams Shea Butter

- 136 grams Castor Oil

- 68 grams Safflower Oil

- 136 grams Fractionated Coconut Oil

- 84 grams Queen of the Nile Fragrance Oil

- 4 grams Tomato Red Fun Soap Colorant

- 6 grams Deep Purple Fun Soap Colorant

Follow the cold process soap making method.

September 14

Lickity Split Lemonade Soap

- 23 grams- Beeswax
- 113 grams- Cocoa Butter
- 23 grams- Grapeseed Oil
- 113 grams- Shea Butter
- 113 grams- Coconut Oil 76
- 23 grams- Avocado Oi
- 45 grams- Castor Oil
- 50 drops- Fun Soap Colorant Neon Yellow
- 56 grams- Lemon Sugar Fragrance Oil
- 172 grams- Water
- 61 grams- Lye

Follow the cold process soap making method.

September 15

Soap Frosting

Are getting creative and making soap cupcakes? Here's a great "frost-ing" recipe!

- 129 grams of water
- 53 grams of Lye
- 21 grams of Almond Marzipan Fragrance Oil
- 170 grams of Palm Oil

- 170 grams of Coconut Oil 76
- FUN Soap Colorant- optional

Follow the cold process soap making method. Scoop soap frosting into piping bags while still warm.

September 16

Whirly Swirly Soap

- 323 grams of Water
- 120 grams of Lye
- 38 grams of Sodium Lactate
- 60 grams of Castor Oil
- 128 grams of Shea Butter
- 15 grams of Mango Butter
- 187 grams of Olive Oil
- 68 grams of Palm Oil
- 255 grams of Coconut Oil 76
- 53 grams of NG Magnolia Orange Blossom Scent
- 12 drops of FUN Soap Colorant Kelly Green
- 12 drops of FUN Soap Colorant Neon Orange
- 10 grams of Titanium Dioxide

Follow the cold process soap making method. Swirl different colors through soap during TRACE.

September 17

Creamy Coconut Soap Bars

- 517 grams Water

- 193 grams Lye

- 612 grams Olive Oil Pomace

- 204 grams Coconut Oil 76

- 340 grams Cocoa Butter

- 68 grams Jojoba Oil

- 136 grams Fractionated Coconut Oil

- 84 grams Creamy Coconut Fragrance Oil

Follow the cold process soap making method.

September 18

Doggy Delight 'Poo

- 172 grams Water

- 65 grams Lye

- 181 grams Olive Oil Pomace

- 45 grams Coconut Oil 76

- 122 grams Palm Oil

- 36 grams Castor Oil

- 68 grams Fractionated Coconut Oil

- 25 grams Sodium Lactate

- 28 grams Sage Leaf Fragrance Oil

- 1-gram Titanium Dioxide

- 6 drops Neon Pink Fun Soap Colorant

- 5 drops Black Oxide Fun Soap Colorant

Follow the cold process soap making method.

September 19

Energizing Soap Bar

- 172 grams of water
- 61 grams of Lye
- 118 grams of Shea Butter
- 68 grams of Meadowfoam Seed Oil
- 54 grams of Grapeseed Oil
- 113 grams of Coconut Oil 76
- 64 grams of Apricot Kernel Oil
- 36 grams of Castor Oil
- 28 grams of Grapefruit Lemongrass Energize Fragrance Oil
- 20 grams of Sodium Lactate
- 4 grams of Titanium Dioxide
- 5 grams of FUN Soap Colorant- Neon Pink
- 5 grams of FUN Soap Colorant- Neon Yellow

Follow the cold process soap making method.

September 20

Frantic Fruit Frenzy Soap

- 517 grams Water

- 199 grams Lye

- 136 grams Apricot Kernel Oil

- 109 grams Coconut Oil 76

- 299 grams Grapeseed Oil

- 476 grams Mango Butter

- 109 grams Castor Oil

- 231 grams Fractionated Coconut Oil

- 7 grams Orange Peel Powder

- 84 grams Fresh Fruit Slices Fragrance Oil

Follow the cold process soap making method.

September 21

Soothing Avocado Soap

- 517 grams Distilled Water

- 175 grams Lye

- 489 grams Avocado Oil

- 272 grams Palm Oil

- 231 grams Shea Butter

- 231 grams Coconut Oil 76

- 136 grams Jojoba Oil

- 42 grams Rice Petals & Shea Butter Fragrance Oil

- Teal Oxide FUN soap colorant

Follow the cold process soap making method.

September 22

Supermarket Soap Recipe

You won't find any fancy ingredients in this soap! Everything you need can be found right at your local grocery shop.

- Water – 11 oz. (300 grams)
- Lye - 4.5 oz. (127 grams)
- Canola Oil – 5 oz. (142 grams)
- Crisco – 8 oz. (227 grams)
- Olive Oil - 11 oz. (312 grams)
- Coconut Oil – 8 oz. (227 grams)

Follow the cold process soap making method.

September 23

Lotus Blossom Sea Salt Soap

- Water – 11 oz. (300 grams)
- Lye - 4.5 oz. (127 grams)
- Canola Oil – 5 oz. (142 grams)
- Crisco – 8 oz. (227 grams)
- Olive Oil - 11 oz. (312 grams)
- Coconut Oil – 8 oz. (227 grams)
- Sea Salt and Lotus Blossom Fragrance Oil – 1.4 oz.
- FUN soap colorant

Follow the cold process soap making method.

September 24

Psychedelic Hemp Soap

- 582 grams of water
- 215 grams of lye
- 413 grams of Shea Butter
- 153 grams of Safflower Oil
- 107 grams of Rice Bran Oil
- 306 grams of Coconut Oil 76
- 245 grams of Olive Oil pomace
- 184 grams of Meadow Foam Seed Oil
- 122 grams of Fractionated Coconut Oil
- 96 grams of Cannabis Flower Fragrance Oil
- 48 grams of Vanilla White Color Stabilizer
- 63 grams of Sodium Lactate
- 6 grams of FUN Soap Colorant Neon Red
- 6 grams of FUN Soap Colorant Neon Yellow
- 6 grams of FUN Soap Colorant Neon Orange
- 6 grams of FUN Soap Colorant Neon Green
- 8 grams of FUN Soap Colorant Neon Blue
- 12 grams of FUN Soap Colorant Ultramarine Violet

Follow the cold process soap making method.

September 25

Wholesome Hot Fudge Brownie Soap

- 517 grams Water

- 202 grams Lye

- 163 grams Avocado Oil

- 136 grams Sunflower Oil

- 408 grams Coconut Butter Deodorized

- 245 grams Sweet Almond Oil

- 272 grams Fractionated Coconut Oil

- 136 grams Macadamia Nut Oil

- 84 grams Hot Fudge Brownies Fragrance Oil

- 42 grams Sodium Lactate

- 12 grams Cocoa Powder

- 6 grams Titanium Dioxide

Follow the cold process soap making method.

September 26

Hunting Trip Super Soap

Attract some game with this fabulous wilderness soap.

- 4.4 oz. Sodium Hydroxide (Lye) (125 grams)

- 12.16 oz. Distilled Water (345 grams) 24 oz. Lard or Tallow–680 grams

- 6.4 oz. Coconut Oil (76 Degree Melt Point) (181.5 grams)

- 1.6 oz. Castor Oil (45.4)

Follow the cold process soap making method.

September 27

Lovely Lady Lavender Soap

- 517 grams of water
- 190 grams of Lye
- 245 grams of Sweet Almond Oil
- 191 grams of Apricot Kernel Oil
- 95 grams of Castor Oil
- 340 grams of Coconut Oil 76
- 381 grams of Mango Butter
- 109 grams of Macadamia Nut Oil
- 85 grams of Lavender Martini Fragrance Oil
- 55 grams of Sodium Lactate
- 1 gram of Lavender Flowers whole
- 15 grams of Titanium Dioxide
- 6 grams of FUN Soap Colorant- Deep Purple (for the medium shade of purple)

Follow the cold process soap making method.

September 28

Girlfriends Soap

- 517 grams Water
- 186 grams Lye
- 408 grams Olive Oil Pomace
- 408 grams Shea Butter

- 272 grams Coconut Oil 76

- 272 grams Palm Oil

- 84 grams Lavender Luxury Fragrance Oil

- 12 grams Deep Purple Fun Soap Colorant

- 24 grams Lavender Flowers Whole Select

- 24 grams Rose Petals Pink

Follow the cold process soap making method.

September 29

Luscious Lime Soap

- 112 grams Diamond Clear Melt and Pour Soap

- 6 grams Agave Lime Fragrance Oil

- 5 drops FUN Soap Colorant Lime Green

- 4 drops FUN Soap Colorant Kelly Green

Follow the melt and pour soap making method.

September 30

Mystic Mango Soap Bars

- 10.6 oz water (300 grams)

- 4.4 oz Lye (125 grams)

- 8 oz Olive Oil (227 grams)

- 6.5 oz Coconut Oil 76 (184 grams)

- 5.75 oz. Palm Oil (163 grams)

- 4.8 Mango Butter (136 grams)

- 3.8 Shea Butter (108 grams)

- 3.2 Castor Oil (91 grams)

- 2 oz. Mango Sorbet Fragrance Oil

- Neon Orange FUN soap colorant

Follow the cold process soap making method.

October

Autumn is finally upon us. I don't know about you, but I'm officially excited. I love the changing colors of the leaves and the spicy smells floating through the air. This month we are going to dive into fall-themed soaps and a few scary ones in lieu of the Halloween season.

October 1

Pumpkin Puree Soap

- 405 grams Water
- 201 grams Lye
- 136 grams Pumpkin Seed Oil
- 340 grams Olive Oil Pomace
- 272 grams Fractionated Coconut Oil
- 136 grams Palm Oil
- 68 grams Castor Oil
- 408 grams Mango Butter
- 3 grams Titanium Dioxide
- 84 grams Pumpkin Apple Butter Fragrance Oil
- 112 grams Pumpkin Puree

Follow the cold process soap making method.

October 2

Nutmeg Butter Soap

- 4.0 oz. Cocoa Butter

- 1.6 oz. Coconut Oil

- 4.0 oz. Mango Butter

- 3.2 oz. Sal Butter

- 3.2 oz. Shea Butter

- 2.4 oz. Lye (NaOH)

- 5.7 oz. Buttermilk (goat's or whole milk) powder in water

- 0.2 oz. Nutmeg Butter (1%)

- Nutmeg essential oil

- Vanilla essential oil

Follow the cold process soap making method.

October 3

Gone Batty Soap

- Clear glycerin melt and pour soap base

- Silicone bat mold

- Black soap colorant

- Licorice fragrance oil

Follow the melt and pour soap making method.

October 4

Jack-O-Lantern Soap

- Clear glycerin melt and pour soap base

- Silicone Jack-O-Lantern mold

- Orange soap colorant

- Pumpkin fragrance oil

Follow the melt and pour soap making method.

October 5

Candy Corn Soap

- Clear glycerin melt and pour soap base

- Silicone candy corn mold

- Orange, yellow, and white soap colorant

- Candy corn fragrance oil

Follow the melt and pour soap making method.

October 6

Monster Soap

- Clear glycerin melt and pour soap base

- Silicone monster mold

- Green and Purple soap colorant

- Sour apple fragrance oil

Follow the melt and pour soap making method.

October 7

Alien Soap

- Clear glycerin melt and pour soap base

- Silicone alien mold

- Green soap colorant

- Lime fragrance oil

Follow the melt and pour soap making method.

October 8

Body Parts Scary Soap

- Clear glycerin melt and pour soap base

- Silicone Finger, Foot, Hand molds

- Peach or brown soap colorant

- Peach fragrance oil

Follow the melt and pour soap making method.

October 9

Icky Eyeball Soap

- Clear glycerin melt and pour soap base

- Silicone eyeball mold

- Blue, white, red, and black soap colorant

- Licorice fragrance oil

Follow the melt and pour soap making method.

October 10

Vampire Fangs Soap

- Clear glycerin melt and pour soap base
- Silicone fangs mold
- White soap colorant
- Lemon fragrance oil

Follow the melt and pour soap making method.

October 11

Creepy Bugs Soap

- Clear glycerin melt and pour soap base
- Silicone bug mold
- black soap colorant
- Licorice fragrance oil

Follow the melt and pour soap making method.

October 12

Slithering Snake Soap

- Clear glycerin melt and pour soap base
- Silicone snake mold
- Green soap colorant
- Sour apple fragrance oil

Follow the melt and pour soap making method.

October 13

Pumpkin Pie Bars

- 20.5 oz. Coconut Oil
- 22.4 oz. Olive Oil
- 18 oz. Palm Oil
- 4 oz. Shea Butter
- 9.5 oz. Lye
- 16 oz. water
- 8 oz. canned pumpkin
- 16 gm. grapefruit seed extract
- 4-6 oz. pumpkin pie fragrance oil

Follow the cold process soap making method.

October 14

Apple Pie Milk Bath

- 1 cup powdered milk
- 2/3 cup fine sea salt
- 1 teaspoon coconut oil
- Apple Pie fragrance oil

Mix all ingredients into a mixing bowl and pour under warm running water.

October 15

Apple Spice Soap

- 18 oz. canola oil

- 8 oz. coconut oil

- 18 oz. olive oil

- 12oz distilled water

- 6 oz. lye

- 1 tbsp. apple pie spice

- 1 tbsp. Turmeric

- 2 tbsps. Apple FO

Follow the hot process soap making method.

October 16

Cool, Autumn's Night Soap

- 8 oz. shea or cocoa butter melt and pour soap base

- 2 tbsps. shea butter

- 1 tbsp. cocoa butter

- 2 tbsps. finely ground oatmeal 1 Tablespoon rose petal powder

- 20 drops red colorant

- 40 drops rose geranium essential oil

- 20 drops ylang-ylang essential oil

Follow the hot process soap making method.

October 17

Red Wine Soap

- 258 grams Water
- 259 grams Frozen Wine
- 195 grams Lye
- 245 grams Rice Bran Oil
- 122 grams Sunflower Oil
- 163 grams Meadow Foam Seed Oil
- 136 grams Castor Oil
- 245 grams Fractionated Coconut Oil
- 449 grams Palm Oil
- 84 grams Merlot Wine Fragrance Oil
- 5 grams Tomato Red Fun Soap Colorant
- 6 grams Deep Purple Fun Soap Colorant

Follow the cold process soap making method.

October 18

Gorgeous Man Soap

- 259 grams of Water
- 91 grams of Lye
- 54 grams of Avocado Oil
- 34 grams Jojoba Oil
- 95 grams Palm Oil

- 136 grams of Olive Oil
- 156 grams of Shea Butter
- 150 grams of Coconut Oil 76
- 54 grams of Castor Oil
- 35 grams of Sodium Lactate
- 43 grams of Total Hot Man Fragrance Oil
- 18 grams of Activated Charcoal
- 4 grams of Titanium Dioxide
- 6 grams of Fun Soap Colorant Tomato Red

Follow the cold process soap making method.

October 19

Sweet Orange Chili Pepper Soap

- 517 grams of water
- 189 grams of lye
- 340 grams of Shea Butter
- 122 grams of Sunflower Oil
- 136 grams of Rice Bran Oil
- 408 grams of Coconut Oil 76
- 272 grams of Olive Oil pomace
- 82 grams of Castor Oil
- 85 grams of Sweet Orange Chili Pepper Fragrance Oil
- 50 grams of Sodium Lactate
- 7 grams of Titanium Dioxide

- 7 grams of FUN Soap Colorant- Tomato Red
- 5 grams of FUN Soap Colorant- Neon Orange

Follow the cold process soap making method.

October 20

Yummy Wheatgrass Soap

- 108 grams Water
- 39 grams Lye
- 51 grams Olive Oil pomace
- 23 grams Castor Oil
- 71 grams Coconut Oil 76
- 71 grams Palm Oil
- 43 grams Shea Butter
- 26 grams Grapeseed Oil
- 18 grams Sweet Grass Fragrance Oil
- 17 grams Sodium Lactate
- 5 grams Wheatgrass Powder
- 2 grams Kelly Green Colorant

Follow the cold process soap making method.

October 21

Lemon Lime Bundt Cake Soap

Shea Butter Melt and Pour SOAP

- FUN Soap Colorant- Brown Oxide 1 oz.

- FUN Soap Colorant- Yellow Oxide 1 oz.

- 7-UP Pound Cake Fragrance Oil

- Silicone Soap Mold- 4 Bundt Cake Molds

- Titanium Dioxide Oil Dispersible

- Veggie glycerin

Follow the melt and pour process soap making method.

October 22

Beet Root Facial Soap

- 380 grams Cocoa Butter Melt and Pour Soap

- 25 grams Vegetable Glycerin

- 12 grams Beet Root Powder

- 3 grams Citric Acid

- Tomato Red FUN Soap Coloring

Follow the melt and pour process soap making method.

October 23

Candy Apple Soap

- SLS FREE Glycerin Melt and Pour Soap

- Wintery Candy Apple Fragrance Oil

- Da BOMB Soap Dye- RED 1oz.

Follow the melt and pour process soap making method.

October 24

Carrot Cupcake Soap

- Goat's milk Melt and Pour SOAP
- SLS Free Glycerin Melt and Pour Soap
- Carrot Cupcake Fragrance Oil
- FUN Soap Colorant- Orange Oxide 1 oz.
- FUN Soap Colorant- Neon Green 1 oz.
- Imagine Base
- Veggie glycerin
- Vanilla White- Color Stabilizer
- Cupcakes- Mold Market Molds
- Embed Mold - Peanut Butter Cups
- Pumpkin Pie Spice Blend Powder

Follow the melt and pour process soap making method.

October 25

Cinnamon Bun Soap

- Goat's milk Melt and Pour SOAP
- FUN Soap Colorant- Brown Oxide 1 oz.
- Cinnamon bun Type Fragrance Oil
- Square Loaf- Mold Market Molds

Follow the melt and pour process soap making method.

October 26

Cammy Clay Soap

Tan layer:

- 120 grams Oatmeal Melt and Pour Soap
- 6 grams Watercress and Aloe Fragrance Oil
- 7 grams Rhassoul Clay
- 11 Grams Vegetable Glycerin

Clear layer:

- 180 grams Diamond Clear Melt and Pour Soap
- 9 grams Watercress and Aloe Fragrance Oil
- 7 grams Chamomile Flowers- German Whole

Follow the melt and pour process soap making method.

October 27

Chocolate Cream Cheese Cupcake Soap

- Yogurt Melt and Pour Soap
- Chocolate Cream Cheese Cupcake Fragrance Oil
- Imagine Base
- Veggie glycerin
- Vanilla White- Color Stabilizer
- Cupcakes- Mold Market Molds
- Embed Mold - Peanut Butter Cups
- Cocoa Powder Organic

Follow the melt and pour process soap making method.

October 28

Ghost Soap

- 200 grams Diamond Clear Melt and Pour Soap
- 1 grams Fun Soap Colorant Black Oxide
- 77 grams Whipped Soap Base
- 77 grams Soya Milk Melt and Pour
- 9 grams Vegetable Glycerin
- 17 grams Alien Type Fragrance Oil

Follow the melt and pour process soap making method.

October 29

Count Dracula's Dentures

Recipe for Embeds:

- 103 grams- Arrowroot Powder
- 24 grams- Vegetable Glycerin
- 112 grams- Diamond Clear Melt and Pour Soap Base
- 14 grams- Fractionated Coconut Oil
- 13 grams- Lunar Eclipse Fragrance Oil
- 3 grams- Optiphen Preservative
- 25-30 drops- Red Da Bomb Soap Colorant

Recipe for Teeth Portion of Soap:

- 24 grams- Red Play Dough Soap

- 136 grams- Goat's Milk Melt and Pour Soap Base

- 7 grams- Lunar Eclipse Fragrance Oil

Recipe for Denture Solution Portion of Soap:

- 788 grams- Diamond Clear Melt and Pour Soap Base

- 39 grams- Lunar Eclipse Fragrance Oil

- 3-4 drops Blue- Da Bomb Soap Colorant

Follow the melt and pour process soap making method.

October 30

Freshly Fallen Leaves Soap

- 1380 grams Diamond Clear Melt and Pour Soap

- 500 grams Goat's Milk Melt and Pour Soap

- 85 grams Fresh Fallen Leaves Fragrance Oil

- 15 drops Fun Soap Colorant- Yellow Oxide

- 15 drops Fun Soap Colorant- Orange Oxide

- 20 drops Fun Soap Colorant- Brown Oxide

- 10 drops Fun Soap Colorant- Red Oxide

- 25 drops Fun Soap Colorant- Tomato Red

- 60 drops Fun Soap Colorant- Kelly Green

Follow the melt and pour process soap making method.

October 31

Monster Boogers Soap

- 69 grams SLS Free Clear Melt and Pour Soap

- 187 grams Distilled Water

- 12 grams Tart Green Apple Fragrance Oil

- 4 grams Optiphen

- 4 drops Da Bomb Soap Dye Yellow

- 2 drops Da Bomb Soap Dye Blue

Follow the melt and pour process soap making method but stop once your soap reaches the jelly phase. Pour soap into a container and decorate with googly eyes.

November

Here we are, at the heart of the fall season. With Thanksgiving just around the corner, what types of soaps can you create to show your appreciation for all that you have? This section will focus on the scents of the fall season and keeping your body hydrated and moistened in preparation for the cool, crisp, Autumn air.

November 1

Star Anise Soap Bars

- 12 Cavity Rectangle Silicone Mold
- 50 oz. Shea Melt and Pour Base
- 13 oz. Clear Melt and Pour Base
- Green Zeolite Clay
- Spirulina Powder
- .3 oz. Anise Essential Oil
- .2 oz. Orange 10x Essential Oil
- Anise Stars
- Cinnamon Sticks
- 99% Isopropyl Alcohol

Follow the melt and pour process soap making method.

November 2

Cinnamon Pumpkin Paradise Soap

- 12 Cavity Rectangle Silicone Mold
- 41 oz. Goat Milk Melt and Pour Base
- 12 oz. Clear Melt and Pour Soap Base
- Perfect Orange Color Block
- Shimmer Cappuccino Color Block
- 1 oz. Pumpkin Pie Candle & Soap Fragrance Oil
- 1 oz. Vanilla Color Stabilizer
- 3 Tbs. Ground Pumpkin Seeds
- 99% Isopropyl Alcohol
- Dash of ground cinnamon

Follow the melt and pour process soap making method.

November 3

Rustic Soap Bars

- 45 oz. Clear Melt and Pour Soap Base
- 1.5 tsp. Crushed Grape Seeds
- .5 tsp. Strawberry Seeds
- .75 tsp. Shredded Loofah
- Desert Red Mica
- Liquid Blue Colorant
- 99% Isopropyl Alcohol
- 1.2 oz. Fresh Bamboo Fragrance Oil (0.3 oz. in each layer)
- Tall 12″ Silicone Loaf Mold
- Crinkle Cutter

Follow the melt and pour process soap making method.

November 4

Warm Ginger Patchouli Soap Bars

- 32 oz. Honey Melt and Pour Base
- 16 oz. White Melt and Pour Base
- King's Gold Mica
- Shimmer Yellow Color Block
- 1.3 oz. Ginger Patchouli Fragrance Oil
- 10″ Silicone Loaf Mold
- 16 oz. Isopropyl Alcohol (99%)
- Crinkle Cutter

Follow the melt and pour process soap making method.

November 5

November Moustache Soap

- Guest Mini Mustache Mold
- 14 oz. Shaving Melt and Pour Base
- Non Bleeding Black Oxide Color Block
- Non Bleeding Brown Oxide Color Block
- Non Bleeding Ultramarine Blue Color Block
- Non Bleeding Perfect Red Color Block
- 3 mL Mahogany Fragrance Oil
- 3 mL Shave and a Haircut Fragrance Oil

- Injector Tool

Follow the melt and pour process soap making method.

November 6

Soap on a Rope Pumpkins

- Spooked Pumpkin 3D Mold
- Spooky Pumpkin 3D Mold
- 9 oz. White Melt and Pour
- Liquid Orange
- Green Chrome Oxide Pigment
- Luster Black Mica
- 2 Black Soap Rope
- .25 oz. Pumpkin Souffle Fragrance Oil
- .25 mL Vanilla Color Stabilizer

Follow the melt and pour process soap making method.

November 7

Shimmering Fall Layer Soap

- 16 oz. Clear Melt and Pour Base
- .5 oz. Spiced Amber Ale Fragrance Oil
- 4 Disk Mold and Package, Plastic
- Shimmer Cappuccino Color Block
- Shimmer Merlot Sparkle Color Block

- Shimmer Sparkle Gold Color Block
- Shimmer Super Pearly White Color Block
- Fizzy Lemonade Color Block
- Neon Blue Raspberry Colorant

Follow the melt and pour process soap making method.

November 8

Save Face Cleansing Bars

- 6 Half Cylinder Silicone Mold
- 24 oz. White Melt and Pour Soap Base
- 2 tsp. Olive Leaf Powder
- 4 tsp. Green Zeolite Clay
- 3 ml Tea Tree Essential Oil
- 2 ml Rosemary Essential Oil

Follow the melt and pour process soap making method.

November 9

Cranberry Seed Soap Bars

- 11 oz Clear Melt & Pour Soap Base
- 8 oz Shea Melt & Pour Soap Base
- 12 ml Cranberry Chutney Fragrance Oil
- 2 tablespoons Cranberry Seeds
- 1/8 teaspoon Activated Charcoal

- Small 9 Ball Silicone Mold

- Medium 9 Ball Silicone Mold

- 4″ Silicone Loaf Mold

Follow the melt and pour process soap making method.

November 10

"The Leaves of Fall" Soap Bars

- 7 oz Clear Melt and Pour Base

- 27 oz White Melt and Pour Base

- Shimmer Copper Sparkle Color Block

- Non-Bleeding Perfect Orange Color Block

- Shimmer Light Gold Color Block

- Non-bleeding Perfect Red Color Block

- Shimmer Cappuccino Color Block

- Non-Bleeding Chrome Green Color Block

- 1 teaspoon Iridescent Glitter

- 8 ml Red Apple Fragrance Oil

- 0.5 oz Arabian Spice Fragrance Oil

- 3 mL diluted Aqua LabColor

- Glossy Silicone Square Tray Mold

Follow the melt and pour process soap making method. Acquire a fall leaves template to help you create realistic looking leaf patterns.

November 11

Licorice Soap Cubes

- 33.6 oz. White Melt and Pour Soap
- 22.4 oz. Clear Melt and Pour Soap
- Black Oxide Color Block
- Non-Bleeding Cherry Colorant
- Non-Bleeding Teal Colorant
- 1.2 oz. Star Anise Essential Oil
- 9 Cube Silicone Mold

Follow the melt and pour process soap making method.

November 12

Pumpkin Smiles Soap

- 18.2 oz Clear Melt and Pour
- Perfect Orange Color Block
- Black Oxide Color Block
- Halloween Pumpkin Mold
- 0.5 oz. Pumpkin Spice Fragrance Oil

Follow the melt and pour process soap making method.

November 13

Honeycomb Soap

- 1 Pound Honey Melt-and-Pour Base
- 4ml Oatmeal, Milk and Honey Fragrance

- 1 Mini Scoop Yellow Mica

- 1 Mini Scoop Honeyed Beige Mica

- 12 Bar Silicone Mold

- Bubble Wrap and Scissors

- Paper Towel and Gold Sparkle Mica for rubbing over the surface

Follow the melt and pour process soap making method.

November 14

Carmel Apple Soap

- 8 oz White Melt and Pour

- 8 oz Clear Melt and Pour

- Flexy Fast Trial Size

- Liquid Brown Colorant

- Liquid Yellow Colorant

- Sparkle Gold Mica

- Dead Sea Salt- Medium Grain (optional for the sprinkles)

- .5 oz Chipotle Caramel Fragrance Oil

- Craft Sticks

- 1 Apple

Follow the melt and pour process soap making method.

November 15

Bath Whip Frosting

- 1 Cup Foaming Bath Whip
- 1 Cup Clear Melt and Pour
- 1 Tablespoon Liquid Glycerin
- 3 Tablespoons Meringue Powder
- 7 ml Clementine Cupcake Fragrance Oil

Follow the melt and pour process soap making method.

November 16

Gnome Soap

- White Melt and Pour
- Clear Melt and Pour
- Gnome Mold
- Gnome Template
- Water Soluble Paper
- Blue Mix LabColor
- Lettuce Fragrance Oil

Follow the melt and pour process soap making method.

November 17

Giving Thanks Soap Bars

- Thanksgiving Mold
- Non-Bleeding Brown, Green, Yellow, Merlot Mica and Liquid (Bleeding) Orange
- Melt and Pour Tool Kit

- Clear Melt and Pour Base

- White Melt and Pour Base

- Pumpkin Pie Fragrance Oil

Follow the melt and pour process soap making method.

November 18

Honey Ale Soap

- 25 oz. Honey Melt and Pour

- Honey Ale Fragrance Oil

- Silicone Tray Pan

- 5 Tablespoons Liquid Soap

- 8 oz. White Soap Base

Follow the melt and pour process soap making method.

November 19

Dainty Little Leaves

- Clear Melt and Pour

- Orange Spice Fragrance Oil

- Water Soluble Paper

- Fall Leaves Template

Follow the melt and pour process soap making method.

November 20

Glitter Cut-Out Autumn Soap

- Scalloped Rectangle Mold
- Slim Broad Rectangle Mold.
- Wassail Fragrance Oil
- Merlot Mica
- Liquid Black Colorant
- Liquid Brown
- Clear Soap Base
- Iridescent Glitter
- Your Choice of Micas
- Leaf Cookie Cutters
- Hair Spray
- Craft Knife

Follow the melt and pour process soap making method.

November 21

Stenciled Glitter Autumn Soap

- Scalloped Rectangle Mold
- Cranberry Fig Fragrance Oil
- Merlot Mica
- Liquid Black Colorant
- Clear Soap Base
- Leaf Template
- Hair Spray

- Craft Knife

Follow the melt and pour process soap making method.

November 22

Realistic Pumpkin Soaps

- Flexy Fast Molding Putty
- Clear Melt and Pour Soap
- Sunshine Yellow
- Fiery Fuchsia
- Sparkle Dust
- Liquid Non-Bleeding Green
- Pumpkin Spice Fragrance Oil
- Butter Cream and Snickerdoodle Fragrance Oil
- Vanilla Color Stabilizer
- Droppers
- Small Pumpkin
- Microwave safe container
- Stir spoon
- Vinyl Gloves

Follow the melt and pour process soap making method.

November 23

Thanksgiving Turkey Soap

- Jelly Roll Pan

- Festive Seasonal Cookie Cutter

- Clear Melt and Pour

- Soap Kit Syringe Injector

- Micas in Fall Colors

- Spritzer full of Rubbing Alcohol (Isopropyl Alcohol)

- Fragrance (suggestions: Pumpkin Spice, Gingersnap, Applejack Peel, Rum Nut Cake)

Follow the melt and pour process soap making method.

November 24

Mother's Love Soap

- Flexible Rose Mold

- Labcolors Canary, Red & Emerald

- White Melt and Pour

- Clear Melt and Pour

- Droppers

- Passionfruit Rose Fragrance & Flavor

- Rubbing Alcohol in a spray bottle

Follow the melt and pour process soap making method.

November 25

Red Lychee Soap

- Clear melt and pour soap base

- Non-Bleeding Pink Pigment (liquid)
- Non-Bleeding Blue Pigment (liquid)
- Non-Bleeding Purple Pigment (liquid)
- Sparkle Gold Mica

Follow the melt and pour process soap making method.

November 26

Ducky Soap

- Melt and Pour Soap Base
- Glass Bowl
- Duck Soap Mold
- White and Yellow Colorant

Follow the melt and pour process soap making method.

November 27

Pilgrim Soap

- Melt and Pour Soap Base
- Glass Bowl
- Pilgrim Soap Mold
- Your choice of Colorant

Follow the melt and pour process soap making method.

November 28

Cornucopia Soap

- Melt and Pour Soap Base

- Glass Bowl

- Cornucopia Soap Mold

- Your choice of Colorant

Follow the melt and pour process soap making method.

November 29

Mayflower Soap

- Melt and Pour Soap Base

- Glass Bowl

- Ship Soap Mold

- Your choice of Colorant

Follow the melt and pour process soap making method.

November 30

Sunflower Soap

- Melt and Pour Soap Base

- Glass Bowl

- Sunflower Soap Mold

- Yellow and Brown Colorant

Follow the melt and pour process soap making method.

December

Winter has come back around and the Christmas season is upon us. For many, this is a joyous time of year. Have fun making holiday soaps this month and even whipping up a few batches to give as gifts to family and friends.

December 1

Christmas Candy Soap

- Melt and Pour Soap Base
- Glass Bowl
- Christmas Candy Soap Mold
- Red and White Colorant

Follow the melt and pour process soap making method.

December 2

Christmas Tree Soap

- Melt and Pour Soap Base
- Glass Bowl
- Christmas Tree Soap Mold
- Green Colorant and various colors for decorations

Follow the melt and pour process soap making method.

December 3

Christmas Ornament Soap

- Melt and Pour Soap Base
- Glass Bowl
- Christmas Ornament Soap Mold
- Your choice of Colorant

Follow the melt and pour process soap making method.

December 4

Candy Cane Soap

- Melt and Pour Soap Base
- Glass Bowl
- Candy Cane Soap Mold
- Red and White Colorant

Follow the melt and pour process soap making method.

December 5

Angel Soap

- Melt and Pour Soap Base
- Glass Bowl
- Angel Soap Mold
- Gold Colorant

Follow the melt and pour process soap making method.

December 6

Guiding Star Soap

- Melt and Pour Soap Base
- Glass Bowl
- Star Soap Mold
- Yellow Colorant

Follow the melt and pour process soap making method.

December 7

Celebration Soap

- clear melt and pour
- white melt and pour
- (non-bleeding) blue liquid pigment
- Champagne fragrance oil
- Milky Way Oval Mold
- Silver Glitter
- Rubber Star Mold
- Pyrex container
- Spoons
- Rubbing Alcohol in a spritzer bottle

Follow the melt and pour process soap making method.

December 8

Gingerbread Body Scrub

- 1 cup of vegetable glycerin
- 1/3 cup of olive oil
- 2 cups of dark brown sugar
- 1 cup of turbinado sugar
- 1/3 cup of cocoa butter
- 1 tablespoon spoon or more of gingerbread fragrance oil
- 5 drops of liquipar oil

Mix all ingredients together in a large mixing bowl. Transfer to an airtight container.

December 9

Minty Salt Scrub

- 1/2 oz. glycerin soap base
- 1/8 cup liquid castile soap
- 1/8 cup sunflower, safflower, or other light oil
- 1 tbsp. jojoba oil
- 3/8 cup Epsom salts (or other coarse salt)
- 1 tsp aloe gel (optional)
- A few drops peppermint essential oil
- A few drops tea tree essential oil (less than the mint)
- Blue or green mica powder for color

Melt glycerin soap base in a double boiler. Add liquid soap & oils. Remove from heat. Stir in salt, essential oils, aloe, and color (mix powder with a little oil before you mix it in). By this time, the mixture should be thick and goopy but still warm. Plop into a glass or plastic container and let cool (or you can use immediately as long as it's thick to your liking).

Source:

https://www.fromnaturewithlove.com/recipe/recipe.asp?recipe_id=264

December 10

Mistletoe Soap on a Rope

- Clear Melt & Pour Soap Base

- Green Mica or Oxide

- Holly Berry fragrance

- Basic Shape mold

- Ribbon or string

- Holly leaf soap cutter (cookie cutter found in kitchen or craft stores)

- Spray bottle with rubbing alcohol

- Blue Mix lab color

- Pearly White Mica

Follow the melt and pour process soap making method.

December 11

Soapy Holiday Centerpieces

If you have made a few of the holiday ornamental soaps from the beginning of the month, place them onto a golden platter or silver serving tray and put them in the middle of your holiday table. This type of centerpiece makes a wonderful conversation starter, and you give dinner guests a little something to take home with them.

December 12

3D Christmas Centerpiece Soap

- 6 oz. Clear Melt and Pour Base

- 6 oz. White Melt and Pour Base

- Emerald Green Labcolor

- Christmas Forest Fragrance Oil

- Various Stars, cookie cutter size (Wilton makes great stackable cookie cutters)

- Flexible Brownie Mold

- Wooden skewer

Follow the melt and pour process soap making method.

December 13

Snowflake Gift Soaps

- Clear melt and pour soap base

- White melt and pour soap base

- Iridescent glitter

- Brilliant Blue Lab color

- Snowflake soap mold

- Fresh Snow fragrance oil

Follow the melt and pour process soap making method.

December 14

Christmas Cooke Soap

- Melt and Pour Soap Base
- Glass Bowl
- Christmas Cookie Soap Mold or various Cookie Cutters
- Various Colorants
- Sugar Cookie Fragrance Oil

Follow the melt and pour process soap making method.

December 15

Christmas Soap Tags for Gifts

- Clear Soap Base
- Brownie Pan Tray Mold
- Liquid Green
- Yellow Mica
- Iridescent glitter
- Merlot Mica
- Red Blue Mica
- Kumquat Fragrance Oil
- Microwave safe container

- Cutting board
- Freezer or wax paper
- Craft knife
- Cookie cutters

Follow the melt and pour process soap making method.

December 16

Gingerbread Man Shaped Soap

- Gingerbread Man Soap Mold
- Clear Melt & Pour soap base
- White Melt & Pour soap base
- Merlot Mica
- Cappuccino Mica
- Gingersnap fragrance

Follow the melt and pour process soap making method.

December 17

Christmas Wreath Soap

- Melt and Pour Soap Base
- Glass Bowl
- Christmas Wreath Soap
- Various Colorants like green, red, yellow. Etc.
- Holiday Wreath Fragrance Oil

Follow the melt and pour process soap making method.

December 18

Christmas Present Soap

- Melt and Pour Soap Base
- Glass Bowl
- Christmas Present Soap Mold
- Various Colorants
- Fresh Balsam Fragrance Oil

Follow the melt and pour process soap making method.

December 19

Fool's Gold Soap Bars

- 23 oz. Clear Soap Base
- Heavy Metal Gold Mica
- Gardenia Fragrance Oil
- Brownie Pan Tray Mold
- Soap Cutter

Follow the melt and pour process soap making method.

December 20

Glitter Snowman Soap

- Slim Short Rectangle Mold

- 1 oz. Iridescent Glitter
- 1 oz. Liquid Blue
- 1 Perfect Red Color Block
- 1 oz. Sleigh Ride Fragrance Oil
- 2 lbs. Clear Melt and Pour Soap Base

Follow the melt and pour process soap making method.

December 21

Glitter Christmas Tree Soap

- Slim Short Rectangle Mold
- 1 oz. Iridescent Glitter
- 1 Perfect Red Color Block
- .2 oz. Shamrock Green Mica
- .2 oz. Yellow Mica
- 1 oz. Woodland Elves Fragrance Oil
- 2 lbs. Clear Melt and Pour Soap Base

Follow the melt and pour process soap making method.

December 22

Peppermint Bark Soap

- White Melt and Pour
- Clear Melt and Pour
- Goat Milk Melt and Pour

- Dark Rich Chocolate Fragrance Oil

- Peppermint 2nd Distillation Essential Oil

- Perfect Red Color Block

- Brick Red Oxide

- Liquid Brown Oxide

- Liquid Black Oxide

Follow the melt and pour process soap making method.

December 23

Lump of Coal Soap

- 8 ounces Clear Melt and Pour

- .8 ounces Liquid Glycerin

- Silicone Tray Mold

- Activated Charcoal

- Iridescent Glitter

- 1 mL Patchouli Fragrance Oil

- 3 mL Cranberry Sweet Fragrance Oil

- Mini Scooper

Follow the melt and pour process soap making method.

December 24

Yule Log Peppermint Soap

- 28 oz White MP Soap Base

- 40 oz Clear MP Soap Base

- Non-Bleeding Red Colorant

- Merlot Sparkle Mica or Bordeaux Mica

- Iridescent Glitter

- Red Jojoba Beads

- Peppermint Essential Oil, 2nd Distillation

- 9″ Loaf Mold

Follow the melt and pour process soap making method.

December 25

Santa Soap

- Clear Soap base

- White Soap Base

- Non-Bleeding Red

- Merlot Mica

- Liquid Brown

- Liquid Black

- Heavy Metal Gold Mica

- 1982 Blue Mica

- Red Blue Mica

- Injector Tool

- Clean Up Tool

- Santa's Spruce Fragrance Oil

- Santa Claus Mold

Follow the melt and pour process soap making method.

December 26

Holiday Ribbon Candy Soap

- Clear Soap Melt and Pour
- White Melt and Pour
- Liquid Glycerin
- Liquid Green Colorant
- Red Blue Mica
- Holiday Candy Fragrance Oil
- Silicone Tray Molds

Follow the melt and pour process soap making method.

December 27

Birthday Cake Soap

For the cherries

- 6 oz. ClearMelt & Pour base
- Perfect Red Color Block
- Medium 9 Ball Silicone Mold
- For the cake
- 46 oz. White Melt & Pour base
- 12 mL Hungarian Lavender Essential Oil
- 5 ml Buttercream & Snickerdoodle Fragrance Oil

- 7 mL Creamsicle Cybilla Fragrance Oil

- Ultramarine Violet Color Block

- Tangerine Wow Color Block

- 5 mL Vanilla Color Stabilizer

- 10″ Silicone Loaf Mold

For the frosting

- 8 oz. White Melt & Pour Base

- 2 oz. Liquid Castile Soap Base

- 3 mL Buttercream & Snickerdoodle Fragrance Oil

- 3 mL Vanilla Color Stabilizer

Follow the melt and pour process soap making method.

December 28

Holiday Bell Soap

- Melt and Pour Soap Base

- Glass Bowl

- Bell Soap Mold

- Gold or Silver Colorant

- Fresh Pine Fragrance Oil

Follow the melt and pour process soap making method.

December 29

Christmas Stocking Soap

- Melt and Pour Soap Base

- Glass Bowl

- Christmas Stocking Soap Mold

- Red and White Colorant

- Cinnamon Fragrance Oil

Follow the melt and pour process soap making method.

December 30

Christmas Elf Soap

- Melt and Pour Soap Base

- Glass Bowl

- Christmas Elf Soap Mold

- Various Colorants

- Vanilla Fragrance Oil

Follow the melt and pour process soap making method.

December 31

New Year's Eve Party Favor Soap Bars

- Clear Melt and Pour

- White Melt and Pour

- Champagne Fragrance Oil

- Basic Rectangle

- Light Gold Mica

- Heavy Metal Gold

- Brownie Pan

- Craft Knife Soap Paint

- 2 parts Liquid Soap

- 1-part Clear Melt & Pour Base

- 1-part Rubbing Alcohol

- 1-part Light Gold Mica

Follow the melt and pour process soap making method.

Conclusion

We hope you've had a wonderful year making your very own soaps, scrubs, household cleaners, face washes, and much more. Always remember to follow soap making instruction very carefully, especially when using lye.

It is our hope that this book was helpful to you on your soap making journey. You begin this adventure as a beginner, and now you're a novice soap maker. Congratulations!

Now, go out into the world and spread your newfound soap-making knowledge amongst the masses.

www.ingramcontent.com/pod-product-compliance
Lightning Source LLC
Chambersburg PA
CBHW071343280526
45787CB00001B/198